Transform Your Body

After

40

A Women's Guide

to

Weight Loss & Fitness

(3rd Edition)

CATHERINE PIOT

Table of Contents

Legal notice

Disclaimer

This book is meant for educational and information purposes only. It is not meant to give any medical advice, diagnose, or treat any medical conditions.

No medical claims are made in this book. The nutrition and exercise advice given in this book will not treat or cure medical conditions, metabolic disorders, or other illnesses.

The fitness and nutritional advice are meant for healthy individuals who want to improve their appearance for cosmetic reasons and not to treat illnesses of any kind.

Any individual with known medical conditions like heart disease, high blood pressure, high cholesterol, and any other disorder, should seek medical advice before beginning any exercise program.

The author is not an MD or RD and cannot be held liable or responsible to any person or entity concerning any information contained in this book. The reader/ user assumes all risks for any injury, loss or, damage caused or alleged to be caused directly or indirectly by using the information contained in this book.

About the author

Catherine Piot holds a master's degree in physical education and gymnastics training and is a Master's Trainer. She has several other certifications as a personal trainer, performance nutrition specialist, and group fitness instructor as well as certificates in massage therapy (e.g., manual lymph drainage, reflexology, energy massage therapy, and Jacobson therapy).

She has over 20 years of experience in sports, nutrition, and fitness, either as a coach, fitness consultant, personal trainer, or teacher.

Catherine has published articles in several fitness publications and operates the website www.catherinepiotinstitute.com, where people find online resources, diet plans, customized fitness plans, and much more.

Catherine specializes in training and body transformation for people reaching their 40s and over. Over the years, she has enhanced this unique ability by working as a professional athlete's coach, strength and conditioning specialist, and school physical education teacher.

Catherine is a Member of the Canadian Fitness Professionals Association.

Preface

I constantly get questions from clients, friends, and family who want to know what I do to stay fit and learn. The idea of writing a book is not something that sprang upon me one fine day - it has been building in my head for years.

I've been in the fitness and nutrition field for 25 years, and that experience has shown me that women have different needs, concerns, and questions over time. I've also noticed that when it comes to training and nutrition, many women don't know what to do or what to eat to stay fit, lean, and healthy.

Many women over forty get confused and eventually give up the battle, only to find themselves overweight, tired, depressed, and victims of underlying health problems. They don't need to feel that way, so I wrote this book.

I want to help everyone who is over forty to change their body, their look, and their lives for the best.

If you are over forty, I can understand your concerns and know the solutions you need. I'm here to show you that you can not only change but transform your body forever.

For consultations, visit my website:

www.catherinepiotinstitute.com

Section 1

40? An opportunity for improvement!

As time passes, biological and physiological changes occur inside our body, and most of the time, we are unaware of them.

We don't notice them at first, but once we hit forty, those changes become visible, and they can be disturbing.

If you are reading this book, you are probably over forty or have a fortieth birthday looming.

Some fine lines and wrinkles may have become more visible; that alone is a red flag. The first gray hair has turned up, and your appointments with the hairdresser have taken on a new urgency. Maybe you feel more tired than you used to, and your joints are stiff in the morning.

However, the worst signs are the extra padding around your hips and belly. Losing weight, even if it is only a couple of extra pounds, is not as easy as it used to be, and you wonder why.

It's a problem, and it is much worse if you still carry some belly fat from earlier pregnancies, which you never managed or even bothered to lose.

Sure, there's a reason for all of this - maybe a demanding job and lots of family obligations - but your body reacts differently than it did a few years back, and that makes all the difference.

Past forty can be a difficult time in a woman's life. The children are older and perhaps have already moved out.

This can leave a huge emotional void, since many women don't feel needed or appreciated anymore. You might be single and start to feel that you are past your peak, or that your dating life is slowing down.

Many women feel like the worst is yet to come because of the menopause and all the associated inconveniences.

But getting a bit older is in fact an opportunity for improvement.

Aging is inevitable. However, this is not all bad! Think of all the new opportunities you will have and of the free time you always dreamed of!

Now is the time to get your life together, get the body of your dreams, and keep it for the rest of your life.

Look at it this way: If you buy a new car and just leave it parked in front of your house without using it, eventually it's going to rust, and the engine won't start.

The same thing happens when we leave our bodies without proper care over time. We start gaining weight and feeling older and tired even though we're way too young for that.

Perhaps you have already started reflecting on your life, on things you did and didn't do, and asking how your life might have turned out if you made different choices.

Maybe you didn't really take care of yourself very well. Or maybe you just took for granted that you have good genetics and eating one meal a day would keep you thin forever.

But the fact is that over the age of forty your collagen production is diminishing, your hormone levels are starting to drop, and your metabolic rate is slowing down. Time passes quickly and without realizing it, you can find yourself looking rounder.

Maybe this losing weight and getting in shape sounds like a lot of hype, and you think I'm crazy. After all, people at 40, 43, 45, or 48 or 55 can't lose weight, right? There are simply too many pounds and for so long...

Wrong. If you think that getting a nice, toned body is a dream, I will prove you wrong!

Instead of feeling down and depressed, eating pizza and sitting on the couch for the whole evening, you are going to start with me, now!

This will be a life-changing decision.

The journey is about to begin, and I will be there with you all the way.

Now, I am writing the third edition of this book, I am 59 years old, and my body looks better than when I was 25.

Why? Because I know what I'm talking about and practice what I preach. And I'm about to show you how to achieve the body of your dreams.

Up till lately, you probably didn't notice weight gain while eating muffins in the morning, a quick but less-than-healthy lunch, a sweet snack at work, and family dinner late in the evening.

Unfortunately, one of the downsides of growing older is that our metabolism is slowly but surely slowing down.

That means that even if you eat the same amount of food as before, you are going to start gaining weight, especially if you are not physically active.

For many of us, gaining weight is a reason to start panicking. Many women think that if they start putting on weight, it's because they've been eating too much, so they assume it's time for a diet.

After all, what seems more logical than eating baby carrots and drinking coffee all day until the weight is off?

But that's precisely what you should not do. It's in fact the opposite of what you should do, and it won't work.

Here's why dieting doesn't work:

When you reduce the calories you consume daily, you will drop some weight, alright.

<u>At first</u> !!!

The trouble is that this **weight** loss is not **fat** loss.

What you are really losing are muscle and water. And at the end of your diet, assuming you can stay on it, you will have lost much more **muscle** than **fat**.

You see, muscles are metabolically active tissues, which means they consume energy and, therefore, calories. Fat, on the other hand, is simply fat.

It's not metabolically active tissue and doesn't participate in the calorie-burning process.

Fat can be used for energy, but within entirely different circumstances and not just by a dieter who want to lose weight.

With a typical diet, you lose what you really need most: muscle. And it's a vicious cycle - when you find you are not reaching your weight loss goal, you decide to cut down on more calories, and your body eats even more muscle!

Why? Because this is our body's survival instinct-mechanism, which consumes energy from muscle tissue when food is unavailable.

When you stop dieting and return to your normal eating habits, the extra weight returns quickly.

You may even gain more.

And that's not all.

More bad news, since you have reduced your muscle mass but kept the fat, your metabolism will <u>slow down even more</u>.

Now you have a slower metabolism, less muscle and a lot of fat, making it even harder to lose weight!

Does it sound confusing?

Well, it is a little. It's also why 95% of the people who go on diets regain weight and end up even heavier.

So far, we have talked about our disadvantages like age, lower metabolic rate, and more fat. Now let's talk about how you must tackle the beast to succeed:

To lose weight you need to be in a calorie deficit.

What is a Calorie Deficit, and Why Does It Matter?

In nutshell, a calorie deficit is burning more calories than you consume. Think of it as your body's financial system.

When you consume more calories (or "spend" more) than you burn, you accumulate "debt" in the form of extra pounds.

On the contrary, creating a calorie deficit is like putting money into a savings account – every day you are "saving" calories, you are inching closer to your weight loss goals.

For women over 40, understanding and achieving a calorie deficit becomes even more essential.

With age, your metabolism tends to slow down, and your muscle mass decreases as we saw before. This means that without any changes to our eating habits or activity level, you naturally burn fewer calories.

To consume fewer calories first you will have to know how many calories you are eating right now. We will see how you can find that out in a short while.

Hormonal changes

Hormones are chemical messengers produced from the body's endocrine system and go directly into the blood.

Hormones have an enormous effect in many important bodily functions like growth and development, reproduction, metabolism, sleep, and mood. What few people know is that hormones are not only affected by aging but also <u>by our lifestyle</u>!

Not only the metabolism is slowing down but our hormones are dropping steadily.

What is of vital importance here, is the fact that our lifestyle and precisely the way we eat is affecting the hormonal system and is the major cause of weight gain. We see now that this happens much earlier and long before you reach menopause.

And I don't only talk about the female hormones but almost every other hormone in the body is affected. Let's have a look at changes and symptoms that you may have noticed and what you can do about it.

Estrogen levels are dropping. Although you still have periods, the drop in estrogen levels can be responsible for gaining weight much more and also for having a hard time losing it. When estrogen levels drop, appetite usually increases.

In fact, you start gaining more fat around your midsection and if you don't pay attention to your nutrition and exercise regime, this will become a real problem.

When estrogen levels drop, your leptin level is also impacted.

Leptin is the hormone that inhibits hunger – If you want, it is more like the satiety hormone.

Another hormone is Ghrelin. This is a hormone produced in the stomach and is called the hunger hormone because it regulates appetite.

Ghrelin levels increase after dieting, which is why weight loss can be difficult to maintain after a crash diet.

To regulate ghrelin levels, especially after trying many crash diets, you must eat small regular meals throughout the day. It will control not only ghrelin levels but also insulin levels. Insulin is the next hormone I need to talk about, and specifically the phenomena of Insulin resistance. Insulin resistance happens when you eat a lot of carbohydrates.

Especially the carbs that are high in sugar and very processed. If you eat lots of puffy cereals, white bread and pasta, cakes, cookies, and other similar foods, chances are you have become or are on your way to being insulin resistant.

The consequence, if you keep the same eating and exercising pattern is that losing weight will be very difficult, but you are probably already experiencing a lot of cravings.

Cravings are the direct result of high carbohydrates & sugar consumption.

More importantly, this habit frequently leads to type 2 diabetes.

The good news, however, is that this can be reversed and corrected with the right dietary changes.

Next are high cortisol levels due to high stress levels. Daily life, family and work responsibilities increase stress levels and somehow turn it into a permanent state.

High levels of cortisol can cause weight gain-especially around the midsection, fatigue, and many other health issues.

Long term stress can literally destroy your hormonal balance and can make you sick.

For example, sleep problems are caused by drops in melatonin levels and high cortisol levels.

We already talked about how cortisol can affect many areas of your life, one of them being the quality of your sleep.

It is the melatonin hormone which is responsible for calming you down and making you sleep.

Unfortunately, Melatonin decreases with age but hopefully it can be taken in capsules and correct the issue.

Quick note: If you have sleep problems, you should avoid working on your computer late at night or check your favorite social media on your phone.

The blue lights of laptops and smartphones make it difficult to fall asleep and have a good sleep quality.

These hormonal issues can be controlled by lifestyle changes and by eating certain types of foods that will bring them to balance naturally.

Using nature's help as much as possible is the best way to give your body the help it needs.

You might ask yourself if you cannot just take hormone replacements prescribed by a doctor.

This is certainly a possibility but usually you won't get prescribed HRT before you start menopause. But even if you can get a prescription, I suggest that you still use the natural option of food.

It's not Menopause.

Everyone thinks that it's normal for women to gain weight with menopause. In fact, it's not the menopause but the drop in hormone levels that make your weight increase. (Hormones do play a role but this is not the first nor the most important cause of weight gain).

Weight gain occurs during menopause simply because we tend to slow down as we get older.

We are less active than we used to be, and inactivity goes along with bad eating habits.

Most women continue to eat the same way after 40 than when they were 30, without realizing the need to change eating habits, because as we already saw, in our 40s and beyond our bodies have very different needs.

Think about it. - at this time of your life you are settled, right?

If you have a career, you might also work longer hours, meaning you sit more at your desk and are less physically active.

You are more likely to skip meals, eat whatever is at hand - or must attend a lot of business lunches or venues where you are "obliged' to eat rich fatty food or even drink alcohol without being able to say NO to anything.

If you are staying at home, your children are probably a bit older and do not need you to drive them around or prepare snacks all day.

You may have less housework.

All of this reduces your physical activity as well.

Those are just examples of how changes can happen without you taking notice. Weirdly, you always feel under pressure, and you keep eating the same way you always did, maybe even more.

So how do you really lose weight?

That's what I'm going to show you. I'm here to help you change the downward spiral and show you that losing weight and having a nice, toned body after forty *is* possible.

As I'm sure you know by now, nothing in life comes to you without effort and there's no such thing as something for nothing.

To get your dream body, you must be proactive. Sorry but you are going to have to work for it.

The good news is that with a bit of effort you'll look fantastic, with the body of a woman at least 10 years younger! If you do not believe me, have a look at my social media, I already revealed my age, and as I post weekly, you can see how my body looks like. (No! No surgeries whatsoever...)

Examine your eating habits.

Before we even discuss how you can get a leaner, better body after forty, we are going to examine your eating habits.

Grab a piece of paper and write down the answers to the following questions (Important: be totally honest with your answers, they will help you realize a few things about your eating habits).

- How many meals do you eat per day?

- Do you have a regular breakfast?

- Do you have a regular Lunch?

- Do you have a regular meal at Diner (Also called supper in some countries)?

- Do you tend to skip one or more of them?

- What does your breakfast consist mostly of? Is it on the not-so-great side like bread, butter, jam, and cake?

- Or is it on the healthy side, with fresh fruit, yogurt, and egg white omelets?

- When you are at work or home, do you like to snack on candy or on whatever else you find available?

- What does your lunch typically consist of? Salads, sandwiches, and yogurt?

- Or Chinese takeout, pasta, fast food, and ice cream? Be precise.

- Do you feel hungry after you finish your lunch and feel that you need a little extra, often sugary?

- Do you have cravings for sweets or other kinds of foods before or after dinner?

- What is your dinner like? Do you eat readymade microwaveable food, or do you prepare your own?

  Again, **be honest** and describe how often you choose these foods.

- What kind of ingredients do you use when you cook? Fresh or frozen?

- How many slices of bread do you have per day? What kind of bread (brown, white?)?

- How many servings of meat and how many fish do you have per week?

- Do you like fried foods?

- How would you characterize your alcohol consumption? How many drinks per week do you have and what kind?

- Wines or beers, or cocktails or hard drinks?

- How big are your food portions? Do you fill your plate with as many things that fit?

- Do you often take second servings?

- Do you often skip lunch or dinner and just munch on chips and other convenient food?

- How often do you eat butter, margarine, jelly, syrups, and peanut butter? Every day? 3 times a week? Once a week?

- Do you eat when you feel down, upset, angry?

- Do you eat when you are bored? If yes, list the kind of foods you eat.

Answering these questions will give you an idea of **how you eat.**

If you answered "yes" more often than "no," you are eating habits are working against both your weight goals and your health, and you should seriously consider immediate action.

MUST: For one week write down everything you eat during the coming week.

Start with your first meal or drink of the day and continue until you include the last meal or drink before you go to bed at night.

This will give you the whole picture of your eating habits.

Often, we are under the impression that we don't eat much or even enough.

When you write it all down you will get a clearer picture of your eating patterns.

For example, if you skip breakfast on most days and on the rest, you eat toast with margarine, you are clearly on the wrong track.

A muffin for example, may look like not much as far as quantity, and a latte is just a beverage, but they are both loaded with empty calories, sugar, and fat.

In fact, you can consume half of your daily calorie requirements just with coffee, muffins, or doughnuts.

If you are an emotional eater and you turn to food each time you have a problem, feel emotionally stressed or even bored, then you need to figure out what is upsetting you.

Maybe you are sabotaging your life without knowing it, because food can provide momentary comfort and we get addicted to it. Unfortunately, it is not an emotional solution.

If you are often at the vending machine buying candy or some other sweet treat, obviously you are going to have a harder time getting in shape.

The point of this little exercise is to make you aware of the quantity and quality of food you eat.

Food can be a great pleasure, but if you want to look better and feel better, and stay that way for years to come, there are certain foods that you must forget, at least for a while.

Better yet, forget that they exist altogether and change your eating habits for good.

Once you come to realize that you not only eat things that are bad choices, have too many of them, and on top of that, drink more than you should, then it is time for a change.

Now, the big question is: how are you going to change?

The real question is how *much* do you want to lose weight, get back in shape and get the best body you could have?

If you want a full change, you can do it even after forty, fifty or later. In fact, after forty, you are mature enough to get serious about it and not waste any more time!

The importance of setting goals.

You've probably heard before that if you want to achieve something, you must want it badly enough. Take it from me - that's not just talk.

Ask yourself these questions:

- Do I want to transform my body, and my life, forever?

- Do I want to change the way I look and feel?

- Do I want to be seen as a dynamic and energetic woman, someone who sets an example for her entire family?

If you answer yes to all these questions, you are halfway there. Now you need to set goals and work towards them. If you want this bad enough, you'll be ready to do whatever it takes to get there.

It won't be easy. On the contrary it will be challenging, both physically and mentally.

Picture yourself five or ten years from today. How will you look and feel if you don't change anything?

Probably much worse...

Do you think you can be happy with yourself, happy with your partner, happy with the way your children perceive you?

In my almost 30 years of coaching women in nutrition and guide them through fat loss transformations, I never met a single woman out of shape that was happy with her situation.

Here are some of the things most of them told me:

-They felt uncomfortable in their body

-They were ashamed of how they looked because they let that happen

-They felt their relationship with their partner had suffered.

-They avoided taking pictures and hid behind other people or their kids when they could not avoid being in one.

-Shopping for clothes was torture.

-They felt worthless because they were incapable of controlling their weight.

-They felt stuck in their career because their weight had started to get in the way of being seen as a candidate for the promotion.

The list goes on and on. Does any of this sound familiar to you?

There is, however, a very important thing to take into consideration. It is something most of us in today's hectic world are forgetting Time! You did not get out of shape or put on weight **overnight**.

It was a slow process, perhaps involving a few years before you even realized it.

Now that you are working in the opposite direction, you'll have to give your body **time** to make changes. Don't expect **overnight** results.

It's important to remember this time element during your transformation journey.

If you want lasting results, then you must do it the right way.

This is not a **quick fix** and certainly not another kind of diet.

If you are here for a quick fix-going on vacation weight loss, this is probably not the right book for you.

This is why I do not believe in diets.

Diets have made the lives of many women even more difficult because they believed that dieting would transform their body.

What they got in the end was muscle loss, more weight gain, a slower metabolism and unbalanced hormones. This perpetuates the weight gain issue.

So, forget about diets. What you need is a road map.

Be specific on how you want to feel, how you want to look, and how much weight you want to lose.

Write it all down.

You have to create a clear picture of where you want to go and how to get there.

It's a plan. All important things in life are planned. You planned where you wanted to go in your career, and if this is important to you, you'll have to plan for your body transformation the same way.

You also must believe in yourself. Just because you are now in your forties and carry some extra weight doesn't mean you can't change.

Of *course*, it is easier to lose weight and get muscle when you are 25.

Even if being older makes physical change harder, it is very doable.

It's as much a mental journey as it is a physical one.

You must be <u>convinced</u> that change can happen. And it will happen.

One way to do that is to visualize how you want to look. If you want to have a flat stomach and shapely legs, then visualize that mental picture.

See yourself as a new person—the person you want to become—then work towards achieving that goal.

Do this little exercise every day: Close your eyes and visualize your success. Then repeat this mental visualization throughout the day and before you go to sleep at night. You will be amazed how this helps.

Repeat often, **"I can do it."** By saying this to yourself, you subconsciously create a positive environment.

Don't underestimate the power of your mind. People have achieved extraordinary things just by believing in their dream and working for it.

Speak to yourself with affirmative words and determine how you want to see yourself.

Set a time limit but make sure it's realistic.

For example, it is reasonable to aim to lose 10 lbs in 12 weeks. Wanting to lose 30 lbs in 12 weeks is not realistic and you'll get frustrated if you try.

You don't have to tell the rest of the world what you intend to do either.

Most of the time, people will criticize you, tell you that you are too old to change physically, become jealous or mean. Just ignore all this and go your own way.

Don't allow negativity and criticism to put you down.

Some people don't like it when their friends undertake challenges.

They prefer that you stay the same, so they don't feel threatened or left out of your new life.

If you suddenly decide that you don't want to hang out with them at the local bar after work, go for coffee and cake, or sit on the couch and eat chips and drink wine, then you are changing their usual scene.

They may feel you are not who you were anymore, or worse, that you are moving on without them.

People may try to sabotage your efforts by bringing food or alcohol around when they know you are trying to change your eating and drinking patterns.

Don't be discouraged by any of this. There will also be people who will compliment and encourage you.

Stay positive. Positive thinking needs to be applied to everything. See the good side of things.

Yes, changing eating habits is hard, but remember you are becoming healthier...

And most importantly remember, you are doing this for you, no one else!

Stay Focused

Always stay focused on your goal. Life is already hectic and unpredictable.

Yes, you may have some setbacks along the way, but the most important thing is to keep your goal in sight and make the step forward.

There will be times when you feel tired, stressed, unmotivated and frustrated.

Things can come up any time, but when you have a goal, you need to stay concentrated.

Don't allow other people, including friends, family, and coworkers, to jump into your life with all kinds of emergencies and take you off course.

This is time for yourself, and you need to make that clear to the people around you.

You'll need to make people understand that you have an important commitment to honor. Especially if you are someone who puts everyone before yourself and really want to please people, it may be hard for you at the beginning to start setting some boundaries.

Don't fall into the procrastination trap either. You must make necessary changes today, not tomorrow, not in a week.

You are in your forties, after all, and you need to do things today.

Remember you can do it. Make a plan and believe in yourself.

Discipline matters

Now that you have set your goals in your mind and in writing, you've already accomplished 2 very important steps.

But as encouraging as it is, this is only the beginning.

For your goals to become reality, you need to work towards them.

This is the hard part.

When it comes to new things, and more importantly, new habits, you often come face to face with our own internal resistance.

It may not be something that you control, but the mind can be so conditioned to certain patterns that it subconsciously resists change.

Condition yourself to do something you are not used to; for example, eat something new instead of your habitual comfort food.

For this to happen you'll have to fight the instinct that tells you to go for the pack of chips instead of the salad, to head to the vending machine instead of eating the fruit you brought from home, or to stay in bed and miss your workout before work.

Discipline is the hard work that comes with goals.

But you must do it if you want to succeed.

You have set goals - now go all the way.

Goals without action become wishful thinking. Magical transformation without any efforts does not exist.

If you think about it, you already have a lot of discipline in many areas of your life:

You wake up every morning and go to work, even on the days you'd rather stay home.

You respect the deadline for the projects you are working on.

You pick up your children from school or respect your commitments with friends or relatives.

You take your medication when you are sick, even though you don't like the awful taste, and you do it because of the goal you have in mind - to get better.

Sure, the whole discipline thing may seem hard at first, but start by taking small steps.

The difference between weight loss and fat loss

We mostly talk about weight loss. However, we really must distinguish between weight loss and fat loss. These are two different things

Let's start with **Weight Loss**

Weight loss is overall body weight. This includes all your body's components: muscle, fat, water, bone, etc. When you see the number on the scale go down, it's often a mix of fat, muscle, and water weight that you are losing.

What is Fat Loss?

We talk about fat loss when we reduce the amount of body fat we carry. Losing excess **body fat** is the **goal**, even when we talk about weight loss.

Carrying too much body fat is not only a matter of aesthetics but of health, since it can cause serious issues such as heart disease, diabetes, and other health trouble.

Why is this important, particularly for women over 40?

As we age, we naturally start to lose muscle mass. It can be something over 5% per decade- a process known as sarcopenia.

This process can begin as early as our 30's and accelerates in our 40's and beyond. So, when we hit 40 and realize we need to lose weight, it's crucial to focus on fat loss, rather than overall weight loss, because we need to preserve as much muscle mass as possible.

How to focus on fat loss:

Now that you know the difference between weight loss and fat loss, here is how you can make fat loss more efficient and long lasting.

1.Strength Training:

Focus on strength training more than anything. This helps to build muscle, which will burn more fat but will also boost your metabolism.

A healthier and faster metabolic rate as we age will allow you to eat more and maintain a healthy weight and a toned body.

2.Eat High-Quality Protein:

As I have already mentioned, protein is one of the most important macronutrients, especially as we age. Eating an adequate high-quality protein in your diet will support muscle repair and growth.

And before you ask, no building muscle will not make you huge not masculine.

3.Once again avoid crash diets:

Most diets restrict your calories to the bare minimum for survival.

Drastic calorie restriction will not only make you incredibly hungry, but it will lead to muscle loss.

Muscle loss is what you absolutely need to **avoid** as you age.

Yes, you need to be in a calorie deficit to start losing weight consisting of body fat but at a steady and sustainable rate of about 1-2 pounds per week.

4.Body Composition is important:

You can look thin and never have a weight issue, but your body composition can be really bad. How can this be and what does that even mean?

Well, your body composition means that your weight is unrelated to what is happening inside your body. You can be lean and still have a high amount of body fat.

High body fat levels are deceptive. This condition can affect not only people who visually look overweight or out of shape, but also slim or visually lean looking.

If you eat high sugary and high fat foods, if you eat junk food and snack on snicker bars, you may remain in a calorie deficit and maintain your weight. But your body composition will be bad.

So instead of relying only on the scale, use other methods of measurement, such as body circumference, progress photos, your clothes size and fit, or body composition tests.

This will give you a more accurate picture of your fat loss progress.

Diet

To repeat what I said before, I don't believe in diets. <u>Diets alone do not work</u> and in the end, you'll just put on weight again.

What I am talking about here is changing your eating habits and exercise regime once and for all.

Let me be very honest with you.

Changing your eating habits will be hard, but you must do it if you want your body to change and enjoy great health in the years to come.

When you know what to eat, what is good for you and what's not, you'll be able to make better choices, and eat <u>more while losing weight</u>.

Once you switch to a new eating regime, you won't feel hungry most of the day, you'll reduce cravings, and you'll increase your metabolic rate.

The substitution tricks.

At the beginning, take baby steps. For the first three days, if you have a sweet tooth, start by deciding not to eat sugar.

Now, when I say sugar, that's not just the sugar you put in your coffee, but you must include everything else that contains sugar.

Forget about cakes, cookies, ice cream, chocolate bars and so many other things that may be on your list of favorites but are full of sugar.

Replace sugar with something else. Let's say an apple or strawberries or even agave syrup.

So now you are going to be eating an apple instead of cookies at work or eating a cup of strawberries in the evening instead of ice cream.

Oddly enough, after three days of self-discipline, you'll start feeling much better and craving less sugar.

You should understand that the more sugar you consume, the stronger your cravings for sugar become, because your body becomes addicted to it.

The greater the amount of sugar you consume, the higher your blood glucose levels rise. This leads to an increase in body fat storage and makes it more challenging to lose weight.

Congratulate yourself for succeeding in this first 3 days tough test!

Now it's time to change something else about your eating habits.

I am speaking of sodas and nachos. Take them out of your diet for the next three days.

The same principle of substitution applies. Replace nachos with celery and carrot sticks and a natural yogurt sauce for dip and drink water with lemon or tomato juice.

It's hard at first, but your body is slowly getting used to the new regime without making radical changes.

Keep up this gradual transformation for two weeks. The two-week adaptation period will help you adjust to your new eating habits.

At the end of the adaptation period, you should be able to execute your plan a lot easier. It will still take discipline, but it won't be as hard.

Discipline is an exercise of the mind. The body will always follow the mind's orders.

From the moment you choose to act about your body and your life, you are on the winning path.

Exercise

The second part is <u>exercise</u>.

Without exercise, no body transformation is possible. Especially for those of us who are way over forty.

Exercise will increase your lean body mass, which is a scientific way of saying "muscle."

Exercise will help you lose weight faster and look much better.

When you have more muscle in your body, you'll have a higher metabolic rate, even when you rest or sleep.

Exercise will help you burn the fat that you carry, and it will tone those muscles that are sleeping and slowly atrophying under fat layers.

And of course, exercise will help you maintain your results.

What I am talking about is how to obtain long lasting results, not the kind that are good for a couple of months until all the weight comes back.

If anyone tells you that you don't need to exercise, he/she is lying to you. Something for nothing? There's no such thing.

What happens if you decide to just diet and not exercise? You'll lose some weight at first - mostly from loss of water - then you will lose some muscle and very little fat, and then you won't lose any more.

When the initial weight loss stops, most people decide to reduce their calorie intake.

Then they lose a little more weight.

The only problem here is that the weight they lost up to this point comes from lean muscle tissue.

Experts have been trying to tell people this for decades: *the less you eat the less weight you will lose.* Why?

When you give your body less and less food for energy, it sees a signal to preserve the energy that it has, since food is no longer available like before. Your body is trying to survive.

The metabolic rate of your body slows down in response to this "starvation".

This protective mechanism is activated every time you starve yourself to lose weight.

You are not losing any body fat, just muscle and water.

The moment you start eating normally again, the weight quickly climbs back up.

The only way to reactivate your metabolic rate is to incorporate exercise.

Exercise burns calories and builds lean muscle tissue. Muscles need energy to function, which means that you will be able to eat more, more frequently and lose weight, or even maintain your current weight and convert your body composition to more muscle and less fat.

Of course, you must increase your calories enough so that your body gets out of starvation mode

See? It's logical!

One thing though, it's important to know where those calories come from, however, and we'll talk about it now:

Let's discuss the contribution of nutrition to a higher metabolic rate and weight reduction.

Nutrition

First things first

First: a good nutrition plan begins with a shopping list. Before you head to the supermarket, take a few minutes to prepare. Don't just buy for a day or two. Make a shopping list of everything you'll need for the week.

You need to make a real plan of what you will be eating during the week.

When you have a list, it becomes easier to stick to your plan. You will tend to buy only what you really need.

Cease the habit of wandering through the store without a shopping list, impulsively selecting items based on what catches your eye. This approach is a recipe for failure.

Typically, what captures our attention are high-fat, high-sugar products that we should steer clear of. Furthermore, these items are strategically placed at eye level for marketing purposes.

Avoid all these temptations. Of course, they taste good, it keeps you full, and you like it, but it's the kind of food that has no nutritional value and is very high in calories and fat.

There are a few things you need to know about these new eating habits.

Once you decide to transform your body, you also need to create a new environment.

Caution: Never go to the supermarket when you are hungry.

When you haven't eaten for a while and hunger pangs are tormenting you, the only thing you can think about is when you are going to eat.

When you go shopping for food with an empty stomach and temptations surround you, you will tend to buy more and your resistance will be nil.

Your hunger drives you to fill your cabinets with all the wrong food, and it will almost certainly sabotage your efforts.

Second: Open your kitchen cabinets and take out everything loaded with sugar and fat.

Scan for items like cookies, cake, white bread, jam, butter, marshmallows, chips, soft drinks, chocolates, and the like.

However, resist the temptation to consume them on your way to the garbage can. It's not advisable to waste food; instead, you can place these items in a box and consider sharing them in the office kitchen, but avoid indulging in them then

Third: Start reading labels. Every single food item has a label that should inform you about the ingredients in it.

Check the list and see if sugar is one of the first few ingredients. If it is, it means that the sugar content is very high, and it's best to avoid this item completely.

Then check the fat content. How many grams of fat are listed?

Remember that fat has 9 calories per gram. You can easily do the math.

Convenience food is usually loaded with empty calories, refined carbohydrates, and fat.

So, when you eat those foods, you are getting mostly fat and sugar and no nutritional value.

Refined carbohydrates will raise your blood glucose level very fast. This level will subsequently drop just as fast, leaving you hungry again.

This is what creates cravings. It's also very unhealthy because it causes you to store fat. In the long run it can even contribute to diabetes.

The right food choices

There are some excellent food sources that can bring your female hormones in balance.

Avocado: avocados are excellent sources of plant sterols that can have balancing effect on estrogen and progesterone. Avocados can also lower cholesterol levels and have positive effect on lowering stress levels by acting on the stress hormone cortisol.

Flaxseed: You have probably heard about flaxseed. **Flaxseed** is a kind of super food. It contains a certain type of phytoestrogen called lignans. Lignans can have both estrogenic and antiestrogenic effects. Flaxseed is also protecting against certain types of cancers.

Broccoli: Broccoli is not only rich in calcium, which is a very important mineral because it supports bone health.

As we age our bones become thinner and broccoli is one of the foods that will support your skeletal health. It also has estrogenic compounds that preserve estrogen balance.

Green like spinach, kale, beet greens and dandelion leaves prevent inflammation, balance estrogen and can also help lower cortisol levels. (We will see soon why it matters).

Soy: Soy mimics estrogen and can help balance low estrogen levels. Drinking soy milk, eating the beans edamame and adding tofu to meals can prevent unwanted weight gain.

Turmeric: Turmeric is more of a spice that you can add to foods and beverages. It mimics estrogen action, and it has anti-inflammatory properties as well. Besides balancing estrogen levels, it can ease pain as well.

Below is a list you can choose from when you shop:

Keep the list with you when you go to the store, at least until the right food choice becomes a habit.

Whole wheat or multigrain bread: (To eat with moderation). Brown, wild, or basmati rice; whole wheat pasta and bulgur. Lentils, chickpeas, beans, green beans, and spinach - fresh or frozen.

Vegetables: your grocery store's frozen foods department has a wide selection of vegetables. Frozen vegetables are almost as good as fresh ones since they are frozen right after being harvested to preserve the vitamins, minerals, and fiber. These take just a few minutes to prepare.

You can buy big bags to keep in your freezer, so you have a variety to choose from, all ready to cook or mix-and-match to prepare in different ways.

Fresh green salad, cauliflower, broccoli (which can be eaten raw or cooked), tomatoes, onions, and peppers are a few good choices.

Fruits: Fruits have high sugar content. So even though it is a natural sugar, it is better to avoid some fruits at the beginning while you try to lose fat.

Look for pineapple, grapefruit, apple, kiwi, strawberries and blueberries.

Stay away from grapes, watermelons and bananas as they are high in sugar. You can have them occasionally and in small quantities.

Remember don't exclude fruit from your diet as they are naturally high in vitamins and fiber and necessary for a healthy diet.

Meat: Boneless, skinless chicken filets, turkey filets, sirloin steak, lean beef are excellent choices.

Avoid processed meat, including lunch meat, sausages, deli- meat and meat products in cans. They are usually low quality and very high in saturated fat and conservation agents that are highly unhealthy.

Always look for visible fat in the meat. Ask your vendor to remove it for you or trim it yourself before cooking it.

This way you will avoid any extra fat in the meat that you would otherwise eat.

Privilege white meat like chicken and turkey (pork is not white meat even though is often considered to be white meat) and less red meat like beef and lamb.

Fish: Fish is a great choice whether you are interested in good health, weight loss, and/or body transformation. You can have any kind of fish you like.

Try to have grilled salmon once a week. Salmon is very rich in good fats. But be careful - if you have it more frequently it can increase your calorie consumption a lot.

You can buy fish fresh or frozen in packs. Frozen is more convenient since one pack contains several servings that can be stored for later.

Cheese: choose low fat cheeses. Sprinkle dishes with grated cheese for a bit of flavor or eat a slice of your favorite kind once a week.

Most cheeses on the market are very high in fat. I know they are tasty, but they are also your enemy.

The good news is that you can have cottage cheese. It's low in fat; it contains a lot of protein, and it tastes good.

Make it a habit to check the labels before you decide. Everything that is marked 45% fat and over is very high and should be avoided.

Milk and dairy: Milk and dairy are generally high in fat, but you can have low fat, skim milk, and yogurt. Fruit flavored yogurt is usually high in sugar and should be avoided.

Go for natural Greek yogurts where you can add real pieces of fruit yourself.

Natural soy milk is also good. Soy milk is very high in protein and helps fight bad cholesterol. Be careful with the different variations. Some are high in fat and contain a lot of added sugar. Check the labels.

In general, use low fat or skim milk for your breakfast cereals or protein shakes. A low-fat plain yogurt is an excellent choice for a healthy snack between meals.

Soft drinks: avoid ALL sodas! Plain and simple. I can't stress this enough. If you can't completely cut them out, have only an occasional soda. They all contain tons of sugar. And zero calorie versions contain artificial sweeteners. Artificial sweeteners of 0 sugar sodas are harmful to your gut, create inflammation and bloating and stop you from losing weight.

Your best choice is **water.** You can add a slice of lemon or a bit of lemon juice to make it taste better if you want or make your own iced tea. Tea and herbal teas are good choices.

What kind of fat can you eat?

Fats have a bad reputation, but some fats are essential for life. In fact, there's a sub-category of polyunsaturated fat, called essential fatty acids, that will do you a great deal of good.

The different categories of fat are: Saturated, mono-unsaturated, and polyunsaturated.

Saturated fat: Saturated fat is the kind that becomes hard at room temperature and is mostly found in products of animal origin.

Essentially the fat in red meat, cheese, and butter is saturated.

Saturated fat of plant origin are things like coconut oil and palm oil. Both are contained in products like cookies and cakes.

Saturated fat, or saturated fatty acids, can cause great damage to health, increase bad cholesterol levels (LDL) and increase the risk of cardiovascular disease and stroke.

Monounsaturated fat: Monounsaturated fat or mono-unsaturated fatty acids are liquid at room temperature.

They are beneficial to cardiovascular health and can lower bad cholesterol levels (LDL).

The best sources of monounsaturated fat are olive oil, avocado, and nuts.

Polyunsaturated fat: Polyunsaturated fat or polyunsaturated **fatty acids** are liquid at both room temperature and when refrigerated.

You will find both in oils of plant origin and fish. They are also very good for cardiovascular health.

Omega-3 and Omega-6, both essential fatty acids, are involved in many important functions such as protection from inflammation of the veins, protection against blood clothing, protection from free radical damage, promote healthy skin and reduce cholesterol (LDL).

The best sources of Omega-3 and Omega-6 are fish like salmon, tuna, mackerel, sardines, walnuts, and flax seeds.

Now that you know the different fats, concentrate on the ones that are good for you.

Here is what you should eat:

You can have healthy fats like olive oil, flax oil, and avocado. You can also snack on walnuts and almonds. The fats you should avoid include fried food, luncheon meats, baked goods, and spreads.

You'll need a bit more preparation and advanced planning, at least until these products become a habit when you buy food, or you cook.

For you to lose weight/fat and to stay healthy, you should try to derive no more than 15% to 20% of your daily calories from fat.

How to eat:

All your meals should include carbohydrates, protein, and some healthy fat.

Until now you have probably eaten 2-3 meals a day. You are probably often hungry, which makes you jump on whatever is handy.

For your metabolism to reach maximum function, the trick is to eat **more often** but in **smaller quantities**.

Remember when you prepared school lunches for your children?

You wouldn't give your children things that are harming their good health and development to eat, right?

So why eat those things yourself?

If you still prepare lunches and snacks for your kids, do yours at the same time!

How many calories per day?

Determine your daily calorie needs.

Once again, to start losing weight/fat, you need less (and better) food and more exercise.

Eating less is generally a positive step, but you need to know how many calories you are taking in to know how much less you must eat.

Note, you should strive for balance, eating less of some foods and more of others, so you can cut calories without feeling deprived.

Knowing how much energy your body needs per day to function is important.

Most of us think we don't eat too much, and yet most people over forty experience slowly steady weight gain.

That's why much of the adult population in the US is overweight, and the trend is increasing in many industrialized countries.

It's a fact of nature that as we age, our metabolic rate slows down.

But that's nothing to be scared about. It doesn't mean that we must eat less and less every year in order to maintain our weight and health.

We can keep our metabolism high enough with regular exercise.

But you must know how many calories your body needs daily to sustain health and lifestyle.

And with some basic information you can calculate your average daily calorie need according to your lifestyle.

For example: If you have a laborious job, you are on your feet all day and you move around, of course you spend more energy than someone who has an office job and only gets up to go to the water fountain twice a day.

Don't get me wrong, every job can be hard.

There are no easy jobs or relaxed lives today. We all have stress. We all feel that we must prove we are still competitive, not too tired, middle-aged, or "passé."

These days, a woman's career journey feels like starting over and over every day.

If you lost your job, finding a new one and starting over again is often like going to war.

This is another good reason to change and take control of your body and life. In a body you love living in, you will irradiate confidence with everything you deal with, work or personal stuff.

Back to calories!

We are now going to talk a little bit about your body's energy needs. Of course, it depends on each individual lifestyle.

Basic Metabolic Rate (BMR)

Calculate your BMR.

The first thing to do is determine your Basic Metabolic Rate,

or BMR.

BMR is the number of calories your body needs per day to perform important functions like breathing, maintaining body temperature, and keeping your internal organs functioning.

Here is a quick calculation to determine BMR:

Multiply your weight in kg x 22.

(For men it's weight in kg x 24).

Let's say you are 130 pounds. To find out your weight in kilograms divide 130/2.2=59.09

Now multiply 59.09 x 22 = 1299.98. Let's round this up to 1300 calories.

This number is your BMR, or basic metabolic rate.

Now, no matter what, your body needs that number of calories just to keep your heart pumping, your kidneys functioning, and your body warm enough.

You <u>should not eat less</u> than that.

This is only the amount necessary for life. You must add the energy you will need to sustain your daily activities like going to work, cleaning the house, working out, driving, cooking etc.

Activity level

Once you know your BMR it's time to determine your own activity level. Here is how to do that:

If you are mostly inactive or sedentary, multiply your BMR by 1.2

If you are moderately active and exercise 2-3 times a week, multiply your BMR by 1.4

If you are active and exercise 3-4 times a week, multiply your BMR by 1.5

If you are very active and you exercise daily, multiply your BMR by 1.7

Let's take case 2 and say your BMR is 1300. Multiply 1300x1.4=1820 calories.

Now you have the total number of calories you need per day. Of course, this is an approximate number.

You may need to add about 100-120 calories depending on the intensity of your activity. Keep in mind that in this case your absolute maximum should not exceed 1950 calories.

In any event, if you consume approximately 1820 every single day, but just lie by the pool instead of exercising, you most likely will gain some weight.

You must adapt your calorie intake to your activity level. Also, you should also eat less on the days you don't exercise.

Remember that the above calculations are maintenance levels.

If you want to lose weight, you'll have to subtract between 200-300 calories from your calculations. Using the same example, (case 2), we'll subtract from 1820. So 1820-300=1520.

Remember that your body needs approximately 1300 calories just to sustain itself, so you'll have to adjust your diet and exercise accordingly to lose weight. You cannot go below your BMR.

Small calorie reductions are better than big ones and give longer term results.

With small calorie reductions you won't feel deprived or hungry and your body will adjust more easily than with big calorie reductions.

Alternatively, you can adjust your workout to be a bit more intense so that you burn more calories.

As you can see, when you increase your activity level you burn more calories, and you can eat a bit more food.

Just be very careful what kind of food you choose.

My philosophy is that especially for our age group, the way to achieve weight loss is a combination of calorie reduction and increased workout intensity.

Fire up your protein intake.

3 things to know.

One: protein consists of twenty amino acids. Two, Amino acids are the building blocks of protein. Three, proteins are composing a big part of our body.

Protein is found in all body cells, muscle tissue, organs, hair, nails, and skin.

Protein is essential to life, to the formation of new tissue, and to regulate metabolic functions. It is also found in hormones and neurotransmitters.

When you first begin an exercise program, your protein needs increase.

This is because your body is using protein to activate your muscles, and because you are eating fewer carbohydrates than before.

Carbohydrates are usually the body's main source of energy, fueling your body with glucose, while fats provide a lasting energy boost once they are broken down into fatty acids.

Proteins on the other side work double duty, aiding in hormone production, muscle building, and protein synthesis.

When broken down into glucose, they become a fundamental source of cellular vitality.

To provide your body with enough energy to function and exercise without consuming the muscle tissue that you need so much; you'll have to increase your protein consumption.

Your intake of macronutrients should look like this:

Carbohydrates: between 40-45%

Protein: between 30-35%

Fat: between 20-25%

These are suggestions and some people do better with a bit higher carbs and lower fat and others do better with a bit higher fat. Very important though, the one non-negotiable thing is protein intake.

In general, I recommend around 1.5 to 2 grams of protein per kilogram of body weight if you are following a program to lose fat and gain muscle.

Another benefit of a high protein diet is that protein contains the amino acid leucine.

Leucine combines with the body's insulin to accelerate the fat loss process while they preserve the muscle.

Remember: to calculate your weight in kilograms, divide your current weight by 2.2.

Now you know how to calculate your daily calorie need, and then also calculate your daily protein need.

Let's say that you are 140 lbs.

140/2.2=63.6 kg.

63.6x2 (protein grams/body weight in kg) =127.2 grams of protein per day

To see how many calories of protein multiply:

127.2x4 (calories/per gram of protein) =509

The best food sources of protein:

To increase your protein intake naturally, you can prepare meals that come from a variety of lean protein sources. Have a look at the list below.

- Turkey
- Chicken
- Lean beef
- Tuna
- Mackerel
- Cod
- Egg whites
- Cottage cheese
- Beans
- Lentils
- Chickpeas
- Low-fat yogurt
- Skim milk
- Soy milk

Note: You must eat protein with every meal and with snacks.

Here is an example:

Breakfast:

- 1 cup whole cereal, or 1 cup oatmeal, or Weetabix, with one cup skim milk
- 1 egg + 1 egg white
- ½ cup berries
- Coffee
- Snack
- 1 protein shake

Lunch:

- 4-5 oz grilled skinless chicken breast
- 1 small mixed green salad with olive oil and lemon juice
- 1 small, boiled potato.
- Snack
- ½ cup cottage cheese
- 1 apple

Dinner:

- 4-5 oz Fish with
- 1 cup mixed steamed vegetables like carrots, peas, broccoli.
- 1 tbs olive oil.
- 1 Greek low-fat yogurt.

This is just an example of how you can organize your menu.

Caution: Avoid all kinds of jams, pastries, white breads, honey, during breakfast.

You can snack on celery sticks, baby carrots, apples, berries, and low-fat yogurt, cottage cheese, hummus, rice cakes, whole wheat bread.

You can also snack on nuts like natural walnuts. Remember, no more than 10 pieces though.

Protein shakes:

Protein shakes are essential and convenient. You should always have one, right after your exercise session. It's an easy way to increase your protein plus, you can mix it with Greek yogurt and berries and make a delicious smoothie.

Always have lean protein with lunch and dinner. Remember, it is better to choose white instead of red meat.

One easy tip: Build your meal around your protein first.

For example, choose a piece of chicken breast as your protein, then choose a complex carb (potato, rice, lentils, quinoa etc.) and add vegetables fresh or cooked.

White meat (chicken or turkey) contains almost no fat. Red meat is usually high in the kind of fat that clogs arteries and raises cholesterol.

Tip: White meat= 2 legs, red meat = 4 legs

Another advantage of protein is that it will cut hunger pangs; you will be full and avoid food urges.

Cravings

Beat the cravings devil!

People who follow restrictive diets often have frequent cravings. So do people who eat more carbohydrates than they should.

Excess carbohydrate intake influences blood sugar levels.

Consuming a lot of carbohydrates causes blood sugar levels to rise quickly, and then fall off just as quickly.

This fluctuation of blood sugar leaves the person feeling hungry and craving more carbohydrate/high sugar & high fat foods.

Everyone gets cravings (not just women).

The problems arise when you give in to cravings for sweets, junk food, ice cream, and other things that you should avoid.

The best solution to that problem is not to skip meals and avoid empty calorie high carbohydrate processed foods.

When you skip a meal, especially breakfast, or when you eat very little or nothing at all, you don't do your body a favor.

After a night's sleep without food, you prolong the period of non-eating until later in the day. While this is not bad if it happens occasionally, it may lead to the opposite effect if you do it every day.

You get hungrier and you are more likely to overeat during your next meal. It's logical, the longer you go without eating, the more your body demands fuel.

This translates into more cravings for calorie-dense foods.

These kinds of foods are high in fat and calories. They include cakes, cookies, candy bars, chips, ice cream, etc...

I am sure you've already found yourself heading for the cookie jar or dig into a chips bag to kill your cravings.

Recent research shows that people who skip breakfast tend to get more cravings and store more body fat than those who regularly eat breakfast.

Since women tend to skip breakfast more often than men, you can deduct the logical conclusion... we are the first victims of cravings.

Many of my clients say they have no time for breakfast in the morning. Another big excuse is that they are not hungry and prefer to wait till lunch.

Not eating breakfast is one of the biggest mistakes you can make.

If you do this for long periods of time you risk losing lean muscle.

Not only do you miss the opportunity to accelerate your weight/fat loss; but you send your body into a devilish spiral.

First it gets fuel-deprived, then hunger hits, then cravings, then overeating or junk food.

Another reason why you don't feel hungry in the morning: it's probably because you ate too much the evening before.

If you have a large dinner followed by ice cream and perhaps cookies or chocolate before bed, then of course you won't be hungry in the morning.

It's normal not to feel hungry after having a high calorie/high fat food right when your body is slowing down in the evening.

Your cravings are most certainly satisfied, but because your body functions are slower at nighttime, digestion takes a very long time.

Since you are asleep for about 8 hours, those extra calories get stored as fat instead of burned for energy.

Then the circle begins again: not eating in the morning, eating very little or skipping lunch, having no energy to do any kind of exercise, and finally overeating at night.

Say stop to this immediately!

Try to eat a little breakfast in the morning even if you don't feel hungry. Some oatmeal and banana or a boiled egg will keep you satisfied until you have your next meal.

If you want to try something different, have breakfast at work around 10, a small lunch around 12 or 13PM, and a snack or the rest of your lunch around 15PM or 16PM.

You will still have energy to work out and have dinner without the usual dessert ice cream or cookies.

Another tip: to prevent cravings and keep your metabolic rate high, eat something before you start feeling too hungry.

Weight loss is about eating right and exercising. Not eating contributes to yo-yo dieting and then gaining all the weight back again.

Now we can discuss the major fuel source of the body:

Carbohydrates

Are they fattening and bad for you?

As I have said before, carbohydrates are essential for good health and physical performance.

Your body needs carbohydrates, and they are an essential food group. It's not advisable to get them out of your diet completely.

Carbohydrates increase blood glucose levels.

When you eat carbohydrates, you can increase your metabolic rate.

Of course, this depends on what kind of carbohydrates you eat and how much. The problems only begin when you eat too many carbohydrates.

Between 40-45% of your calories should come from carbohydrates as we saw earlier.

When you eat carbohydrates, they are either stored as glycogen or as fat. If they are stored as glycogen, they can be used later for energy.

However, if you consume too many carbohydrates and you don't do enough physical activity, blood glucose levels rise quickly and then the carbohydrates are stored as fat.

There are two kinds of carbohydrates: Starchy and complex.

We categorize foods that raise insulin level fast and are easily stored as fat as **starchy carbohydrates**.

For example, candies, cake, fast food, and all forms of processed food.

Complex carbohydrates, on the other hand, keep you full longer. Because they need more time to break down and get digested.

So, they provide energy for much longer and they don't leave you hungry too soon after a meal.

We categorize foods like green beans, kidney beans, lentils, cheek peas, broccoli, spinach, tomatoes, lettuce, and whole wheat bread, as **complex carbohydrates**.

You should consume <u>mostly complex carbohydrates</u> and <u>avoid starchy carbohydrates</u>.

Complex carbohydrates rank high on the Glycemic Index. Let's have a look at the Glycemic Index.

Glycemic Index

What is the Glycemic Index?

The Glycemic Index (GI) is a method of ranking the different carbohydrate foods according to their tendency to raise blood glucose levels.

The GI ranking is based on a 100-point system. Any food ranked 70 and above is called "high glycemic."

56 to 69 are ranked "medium glycemic" and 55 or below are "low glycemic".

Those that raise blood glucose levels quickly are ranked high in the index.

Those that raise blood glucose levels slowly are ranked low in the index.

Ironically, carbohydrates with low rankings are the best ones to eat. They break down slowly and provide energy for a long time.

Carbohydrates that are low on the glycemic index are the key to energy, permanent weight loss, and good health.

You should focus on eating foods ranked medium or below. Your best choices will be in the lower ranking.

For example, green beans and lentils rank low in the index.

White bread, bagels, and cake rank high.

As a rule of thumb, almost all green vegetables (like beans, broccoli, cauliflower, and lettuce) rank low.

So do basmati rice, brown rice, lentils, quinoa, tomato, apples, and kiwi.

All high sugar, highly processed foods rank high.

These can not only make you fat but may also damage your health, cause diabetes or high blood pressure, and clog your arteries.

To lose weight, stay away from them.

How to calculate your daily carbohydrate demand

In the previous section I showed you how to calculate your daily calorie requirement according to your Basic Metabolic Rate and your activity level.

Now let's say that you are a 145 lbs. woman who is moderately active.

Divide 145lbs/2.2 = 65.9 kg x 22 = 1450 calories x 1.4 for activity level=2030 calories per day.

If you get 50% of your daily calories from carbohydrates, then multiply: 2030x .5 = 1015 calories

Now to find out how many grams of carbohydrates you should eat, do the following calculation:

1015/4 (calories per gram of carbohydrate) =253.75

Then divide 253.75 by the number of meals you eat per day, you'll see how many carbohydrates you should have per meal.

Now, if you want to lose weight, multiply your ideal weight by the activity level and divide it by the percentage of your daily carbohydrate intake.

Example: 61.4 kg x 22= 1350 x 1.4 = 1891

1891 x .5 = 945.5 calories

Carbohydrates have 4 calories per gram. To calculate how many calories from carbohydrates you should eat, divide your number by 4.

945.5/4=236.37 grams

Remember: don't try to reduce calories drastically. Small changes bring long-lasting results.

Dietary fat will make you fat.

Fat has far more calories than carbohydrates and protein, which both have 4 calories per gram; remember, fat has calories per gram.

The problem with fat is that when you eat it, you don't feel satisfied right away.

Most likely you consume too much fat. High fat foods are also high calorie foods.

The only fats you should eat are those coming from omega3 and omega 6 fatty acids.

The best sources of omega 3 and omega 6 are fish like salmon and mackerel, nuts like walnuts and flax seeds.

Some things you should know about food:

- Canned fruit, salad dressings, and ketchup are loaded with sugar.

- If you eat foods that are high in fiber, you will feel fuller. Such foods are whole grains, vegetables, and fruits.

- If you are hungry before having your dinner, eat a salad, a piece of fruit or a small serving of soup before your main dish. This will decrease your appetite and reduce your total calorie intake while increasing fiber and vitamins.

- You can allow yourself one cheat day per week. If you are an ice cream lover, allow yourself one ice cream day per week to enjoy your favorite treat.

But remember not to overindulge. One serving should be your limit.

And leave out all the extras that come with it!

Also:

- Don't skip meals.

- Plan your day in advance and prepare meals and snacks to take with you if you work long hours, shifts, or if you travel.

- Plan not only your main meals but also your small snacks throughout the day.

- Plan almonds and walnuts or cup of yogurt, for emergency hunger pangs.

- When at work, try to take regular breaks, so you can refuel with a snack and not go too long without food. This will accelerate your metabolism and give you more energy.

- Plan and prepare your meals for the week and then store them in containers so you have them ready to grab and go or heat and eat.

- If you must eat a lot in restaurants due to business obligations, choose low fat dishes with lots of vegetables. Go for tomato sauce instead of those high fat mayonnaise or white sauces.

- Avoid desserts that are high in sugar and choose fruit salads or sorbet instead of ice cream.

- Of course, moderate your alcohol consumption.

The importance of water

The human body is composed of roughly 60-70% water. All our organs contain water.

Our muscles, our brain, even our lungs, all need water. Our blood contains water. Water is vital in regulating body temperature and transporting nutrients.

It also carries oxygen to cells, lubricates the joints, and removes waste.

Drinking enough water is very important, especially when you exercise.

Sweat and respiration deplete your body's water and you need to replace the lost amounts.

You need to drink around a ½ gallon over the course of the day.

Don't wait until you are thirsty. Feeling thirsty may mean that you are already dehydrated.

During exercise, always have water with you and drink it regularly in small sips.

If you tend to drink a lot of coffee during the day you need to be especially careful. Coffee is a diuretic and causes water to leave your cells.

Always keep water available at work or when you travel.

Drinking water keeps your mind sharp; your body hydrated and helps control your appetite.

Try to drink half a glass of water before every meal.

It will regulate hunger so you will eat slower and avoid overeating.

Water will help with your weight loss because it flushes the byproducts of fat breakdown out of your body faster.

Sodas are different from water. You may think that they help to satisfy your liquid requirements, but sodas contain sugar or sugar substitutes, and many other chemicals.

They give you a lot of extra calories. Exactly what you should avoid. They cause bloating and have no nutritional value whatsoever.

On the contrary, water has no calories and is healthy, so you definitively switch to water (ideally still water).

You can add flavor to your water by inserting a slice of lemon in your glass or a bit of lemon juice in your water bottle.

That will give you the taste and some extra vitamin C.

Another great reason to drink water is that, as we age and our hormonal changes increase, drinking water keeps our skin hydrated and balanced.

Water will maintain tissue hydration and your skin will look moisturized and full of elasticity.

On the contrary, if you don't drink enough water, your skin will look old, tired, dehydrated.

Quite the opposite of what we want.

Exercise

In addition to maintaining a healthy diet and proper hydration, the second crucial pillar of our journey to shed excess weight and achieve a transformative body lies in one essential factor: regular exercise.

What kind of exercise you should do?

You must do cardio exercises and resistance/weight, training.

You don't have to run or jump for hours. Depending on your current condition, on how much body fat you carry, and on your goals, you will need to have at least two to three 20-30 minutes cardio sessions per week.

Doing cardio is not only important for burning fat, but also excellent for maintaining good cardiovascular health. Taking care of our heart and arteries is especially important for people over 40 and +.

Your cardio sessions will achieve just that and will also keep cholesterol and triglycerides (factors of increased cardiovascular diseases risk) under control.

Cardio sessions can include:

walking and jogging, either on a treadmill or outdoors, cycling inside or outdoors, using elliptical or step machines, jumping ropes, or running upstairs.

These are possibilities you can mix and match. Decide and make it fun.

Depending on your end goals, you may have to do 20-45 min of cardio 3-5 times a week.

You don't need to be fast or jump nonstop. Speed is not important.

A slower pace will be easier on you and is better for fat loss.

You can use intervals of fast walking and jogging, uphill walking on the treadmill, and light jogging.

You don't have to obsess with cardio. Don't spend every single minute running or biking.

Avoid over-training; it doesn't necessarily mean that you will get faster or better results.

If weight loss/fat loss is one of your objectives, the way to go is to eat better quality food and less of it, along with cardio sessions and weight training.

What can happen if you don't exercise?

With our way of life today even young women are experiencing serious weight problems.

Don't let this be your excuse to continue an unhealthy lifestyle.

Now, after forty, with our slower metabolism, it's not only more difficult to get back on track, but the health risks are considerably higher.

That's why you should take action <u>now</u>.

Unknown to many, women are prone to the same diseases as men: heart attacks and strokes are no longer just male diseases.

If you carry extra pounds over a long period of time and if your eating habits are not great, then you probably have some clogged arteries or arteriosclerosis.

Even if you don't, high cholesterol, triglycerides, and high blood pressure await you.

Most people - men or women - take medication at some point in their lives to control these diseases and for others that derives from them.

According to statistical data from the American Diabetes Association, 19 million Americans are diabetic; 79 million are in pre-diabetic condition; 7 million have the disease without knowing it; and almost 2 million new cases are estimated every year. The same trend is observed in many countries.

Diabetes has a direct link to extra weight and obesity.

It also has direct links to heart disease and stroke, kidney disease, high blood pressure, blindness, and of course early death.

Now, if you think about the enormous costs of treatments and medication for these diseases, it is scary.

The good news is that this is almost entirely preventable. By taking care of your weight and your health, you will feel much better and safer.

Let me tell you about a client of mine, who at 70 years old finally decided to take control of her life.

Here is how she reversed the situation:

Sophia was 20 lbs. overweight and at age 70 the diagnosis fell like an axe: advanced diabetes.

Until then she wasn't even aware, she had it. She was feeling great and was even very active for her age.

Suddenly she had to inject insulin daily.

When I first told her that her condition could be controlled with diet and exercise, she thought it was impossible at her age.

But when she made up her mind and had the discipline to follow through, she got results.

She loved good food, and she didn't want to pass on the different social invitations that she received 2-3 times a week.

So, for a while she continued the same old way, eating all her favorite foods and taking insulin.

Until one day something changed.

She decided that she didn't just want to give up and wait for the disease to worsen to irreversible conditions.

She started an exercise program by walking 4 miles a day. She also finally started to eat reasonably.

She basically cut out fatty foods, bread, and sweets.

In three months', time, she dropped the 20 lbs. she had been carrying around for at least 15 years and her diabetic condition improved so much that she didn't even need the insulin injections anymore!

She couldn't believe it.

She feels great now. In fact, she told me that if she had realized that she was going to feel so good she would have done it a long time ago.

It is never too late to turn your life around and be the best you can at any age. If she could do it at 70, so can you at 40.

How to make time for exercise with a busy schedule

Life is very busy for most of us. There is hardly anyone out there sitting at home on the couch only taking care of the things they should do to lose weight.

Women are usually juggling many hats at the same time from career to family and everything in between.

The truth is we all have the same 24 hours in a day. It is not a question of finding the time rather than making the time for something that is important to you.

#1 Make it a priority: Exercise is important not only for you to lose weight, but also, for your overall and mental health.

Plan it in your calendar, write it down on your to do list and schedule a time that you can do it.

This may be early in the morning, which means that you will have to sacrifice a bit of sleep, or after work or in your midday break. You can work things around as long as this is a priority for you-and it should be.

#2 Use the breaks: We all take small breaks during the day. If you work in an office and tend to take several short breaks, use them to be active: take a brisk walk or do some exercises at your desk.

You can do some leg exercises like squats, kickbacks, split squats etc. without even leaving your office. You can even do ab exercises from standing position or even when sitting in your chair.

These short exercise breaks add up to your daily activity and calorie expenditure. It means you burn more calories, and you will definitely feel more energized.

#3 Create the habit: the more you do something, the easier it gets. You need to include exercise in your schedule until it becomes a part of your life.

Your body will start feeling the need to do it and it will become easier and easier.

#4 Use time wisely: If you don't have a whole hour to dedicate to a workout, you can either split your workouts into 2 x30 min or you can try doing circuits and HIIT.

(HIIT stands for High-Intensity Interval Training. It is a popular and effective fitness training method that involves alternating short bursts of intense exercise with brief periods of rest or lower-intensity activity).

HIIT workouts are designed to push your body to its limits during the high-intensity intervals, which typically last for 20 to 60 seconds, followed by a recovery period that can range from 10 seconds to a minute or more.

You will be done in no time, and you will get an intense and very effective workout without having to use heavy weights or multitude of machines.

#5 Get some basic equipment for your home: You can get a good workout at home just by getting pairs of dumbbells, resistance bands and a bench.

Most exercises can be done with these basic things. Even without the time to get to the gym you can get a decent workout at home.

#6 If you have a friend or family member who would like to join you in your workouts, embrace it, because it is a great way to hold each other accountable and keep motivated.

Often workout buddies create a healthy competition with each other, and this is mutually beneficial.

And remember, having a coach is the best way to keep you accountable and on track.

Then what to do next?

Next, you need to engage in a weight-training program.

Lifting weights is not going to make you huge, if you are worried about that.

Women don't have the physical ability to do that, unless they take steroids.

Men can develop big muscles with hard training because they carry the anabolic hormone testosterone, which is responsible for masculine characteristics like muscle development.

Women carry testosterone in their bodies as well, but in small quantities that don't allow that kind of muscle development.

However, even for a woman, lifting weights will help your body burn fat quicker and you'll accelerate the fat burning mechanism.

As I mentioned before, weight training gives you more muscle mass, it wakes you up and activates the muscle you have under the layers of fat.

Also, weight training accelerates your metabolism because the working muscles need to be sustained. When you exercise, they consume more of the energy that comes from both food and stored fat.

But be warned, it is not because you start or increase exercising that you can indulge in eating everything again.

Stuffing yourself with cookies after training is not going to be used as energy for your muscles, nor will it make you lean. It will be stored as fat, and all your effort at the gym will be for nothing.

You might even see your weight increase, which will frustrate you a lot.

However, with the right food selection, you can turn your body into a fat burning machine and what you will like most is the way your body responds to resistance training.

You will start seeing defined muscles in places you did not even know existed. Your body shape will change, and you will feel a million times better, both physically and mentally.

You will observe changes very soon after starting a resistance program.

What better motivation is there than seeing actual results? However, remember this is not a **one-week journey**. You must give it **time** and be patient.

The good news is that you don't have to lift weights more than 4 times a week. I will give you exercises and programs that you can follow.

You can also add different variation of exercises once you know how to do them right.

How much resistance should you use?

The resistance you choose should be heavy enough to challenge your muscles, but not so much that it gets difficult to perform the exercise the correct way.

If you have done sports or worked out in the past, you probably have some base line of muscle.

Select a weight that allows you to complete the specified number of repetitions while maintaining good technique. Initially, your main focus should be on performing the exercises correctly.

For upper body exercises, consider starting with 12-15 repetitions, and for lower body exercises, you can begin with up to 20 repetitions.

Learn what you don't know instead of opting for a heavier weight and performing the exercise incorrectly.

Take the time to do the movement without any weight at first, so that you get the feeling of how you should do it when you use weight.

Remember that you are not competing with anybody but yourself.

We all started in the same place, with little or no knowledge at all. So, take the time to learn and don't be afraid or embarrassed to ask if you don't know how to do an exercise.

Being willing to learn and take the next step is what makes a difference.

If you need to improve muscle tone in certain parts of your body more than others, you can work with a heavier weight that allows you to do 8-10 repetitions.

For example, if you want rounder shoulders, pick a slightly heavier weight when doing shoulder exercises. This range will challenge your muscles enough for muscle growth.

Careful, this weight range should only be used once you master the basics. If you are just starting and have never worked out with weights before, it's more important to learn the proper way of executing the exercises.

Learning the basics will give you a foundation for growth and prevent you from injuring yourself.

Resistance training is not only highly recommended for people who want to build muscle, but also for the elderly population.

Although we are not in this category yet, a women's body goes through a lot of changes in a lifetime.

Hormonal changes, pregnancies, and menopause weaken bones and make them brittle.

Weight training strengthens bones and protects them from osteoporosis.

Many studies have shown that older woman in early stages of osteoporosis show very good results in regaining bone mass and reversing osteoporosis, once they start a weight training.

This alone is a great reason to take up weight training today.

Remember, weight training should be combined with proper nutrition. If you exercise intensely at the gym but follow it up with unhealthy meals like fast food and late-night ice cream, you are unlikely to see significant improvements in your physique; in fact, you may experience the opposite outcome.

The same principle applies to nutrition – even if you eat well with plenty of fruits and vegetables, if you treat the gym as a social event and take long breaks between exercises, you won't make much progress when it comes to achieving a toned and transformed body.

Small effort, small results

You must be honest with yourself. Just going to the gym and spending a couple of hours talking to the people you know without breaking a sweat is unproductive.

If you decide to make changes, then be serious about it and commit your time to doing it right. I don't say this to discourage you; I only want to give you the truth and the right facts.

You need to recognize that this journey is entirely your own. The power to undergo this transformation lies solely within you.

When you are in your forties, it's true that you may need to put in more effort than a 25-year-old, but remember, "hard" is not synonymous with "impossible."

Throughout my years, I've witnessed numerous women well into their forties attain remarkable physiques. What united them all was unwavering dedication and an unquenchable thirst for change.

You possess the same potential for greatness. You can do this too. Embrace the challenge and watch yourself soar.

It is time to start your journey.

If you are reading this and have made the powerful decision to embark on a transformation journey, it's likely that you are not entirely content with the reflection in the mirror or how your clothes fit at this moment.

Remember, significant change doesn't occur overnight, and it may not be immediately visible to you. To truly gauge the transformation, you are undergoing in your appearance, the most effective approach is to meticulously document your progress.

This record will be your tangible proof of the remarkable journey you are on. Keep going; every step forward is a step closer to your goals.

Start by weighing yourself. You need to determine your exact weight before you begin. Knowing your starting point is essential to track your progress and measure your achievement against your goals.

If you already have a gym membership, you can request a body fat measurement. Knowing not only your weight but also the percentage of that weight that is fat is even more valuable.

Here's a secret: Many times, when you don't see the numbers on the scale decrease, it's not because you haven't lost any fat, but because you have gained muscle through your training.

Afterward, I recommend taking a full-body picture of yourself, preferably in a bathing suit or underwear.

Pictures never lie.

You don't have to show the picture to everybody, just someone you trust: a husband, partner, or friend. Otherwise just keep it to yourself.

You may not like what you see, but sometimes shock therapy brings positive results.

People don't always tell you the truth when you ask them if they think that you have put on weight.

From their point of view, by letting you believe everything is fine they keep the peace, and your feelings are not hurt. Besides it's not easy to say to someone - especially a woman - "You have put on weight. You should do something."

The point of taking a picture of yourself is to look at it regularly and remind yourself that you have a mission to accomplish because you don't like what you see right now.

Home exercise or gym?

Having some equipment at home can be incredibly useful. Perhaps you have an old bench and unused dumbbells stowed away in your basement?

For a start, these can work just fine. It's better to kickstart your fitness journey with the equipment available to you right now, rather than waiting until you can afford to invest in the perfect home gym setup or an expensive gym membership.

If you are already a member of a gym, that's fantastic. Gyms typically offer a wide array of quality equipment, allowing you to perform a variety of exercises and variations. However, even if you regularly visit a gym, I still recommend maintaining some basic equipment at home.

Depending on available space, maintaining a few essentials, such as dumbbells, an exercise mat, an exercise ball, and perhaps a treadmill or stationary bike, is a wise choice.

This approach ensures you're equipped to perform your exercises, regardless of circumstances.

Ensuring these items are readily available facilitates the consistent maintenance of your workout routine. Should you find yourself pressed for time or unable to visit the gym, the convenience of home equipment allows you to easily modify your workout for a quick and intense session on the spot.

If investing in a treadmill or stationary bike isn't feasible, consider outdoor alternatives for your cardio workouts. Activities like jogging, bicycling, skating, and power walking can be excellent choices.

However, it's important to acknowledge that these outdoor activities are weather-dependent, and extreme conditions can disrupt your workout schedule. Weather can become a factor that affects your progress and sometimes serves as a tempting excuse to skip workouts, not only on bad weather days but also when you are feeling lazy or just not in the mood for exercise.

Stay committed to your fitness goals, and remember, adapting to different conditions is part of the journey.

I also recommend that you invest in a good workout program – made for you by a trainer- so you can get exercise at home when the weather doesn't allow you to exercise outside.

For quick and effective workouts, items like elastic bands and TRX suspension training can be highly beneficial. A TRX (Total Body Resistance Exercise) is a form of resistance exercise that utilizes a system of ropes, known as TRX straps, and will allow you to work against your own body weight. It's designed to develop strength, balance, flexibility, and core stability simultaneously.

In contrast, Gyms provide a wide selection of equipment and exercise options, offering you access to numerous tools and facilities including cardio equipment, dumbbells, barbells, and various machines. They enable a more rigorous workout by facilitating exercises that may be unachievable with your limited home equipment.

A dynamic, lively gym atmosphere and the visibility of others exercising can act as robust motivation. Observing the determination of women, who, despite busy schedules, jobs, and additional responsibilities, prioritize their fitness goals, can serve as a significant motivational boost.

Choosing to utilize both a gym membership and home equipment, if you can afford it financially, is advantageous. This approach allows you to follow a diversified and flexible fitness routine, leveraging the benefits of both environments.

Don't forget your journal.

To attain your weight loss and body transformation objectives, further modifications to your approach are necessary. If you had previously attempted weight loss without success and couldn't determine why, this time, you will adopt a new strategy by meticulously documenting your journey.

Start by getting a notebook and use it to record various aspects of your journey. Begin with measurements of your body. While a professional should ideally measure your body fat percentage, you can assess your waist, hips, arms, and chest.

Make sure to record the date of each measurement. Additionally, specify your weight and measurement goals.

Carry this journal with you during your workouts so you can document your exercise routines accurately. The same goes for your dietary habits.

An alternative and convenient method is to use a dedicated app. Many apps allow you to log your food intake and provide detailed information about macronutrients (carbs, protein, and fat) — a valuable tool for reaching your daily nutritional goals.

I personally recommend using MyFitnessPal as it's user-friendly, features a vast food database, and offers a free version suitable for your recording needs.

Every time you consume something, whether it's a small bite, a shake, or a supplement, record it in your journal or the app. This practice ensures that you have a precise record of your dietary intake, including what you eat, how much, and when.

Also, consider documenting your emotions. Recognize any patterns related to emotional eating, such as reaching for food when feeling down or upset. This awareness can help you prevent emotional overeating.

Having a comprehensive overview of your workout and dietary plan is crucial for making progress. Often, to move to the next level, you may need to make adjustments or changes.

Having all the data at your disposal is the key to finding effective solutions and continuously advancing toward your goals. Besides it is another exercise in discipline, as you must write down everything.

Exercise process

Always begin your exercise routine with **a warm-up**, whether it's cardio or weight training. Warming up your muscles is **<u>crucial</u>** to prevent injuries and prepare your body for the upcoming workout. Include a cardio session in your daily workout.

At our age, we tend to gain weight easily and retain it. Therefore, it's prudent to engage in some form of cardio 3-4 times a week. This could be a simple activity like walking or biking; it doesn't have to be exhausting, but it should elevate your heart rate.

Doing between 20-30 minutes per session should be your goal.

If you find it hard to do 30 min straight at first, break it in half.

Do 15 minutes of treadmill and then go straight to an elliptical trainer for another 15 minutes if you do this at the gym.

If you are a very busy person do 10 min of brisk walking in the morning, during lunchtime and in the evening.

If you already have enough stamina, go for 30 straight minutes of your favorite cardio exercise.

Your aim is for cardiovascular conditioning and fat loss. That's very important so don't cut it short.

Depending on your weight loss goal, you will have to eventually change your cardio time. Slight increases in time or intensity may be necessary to break plateaus and accelerate fat loss.

Weight training

Weight training is necessary for every woman. Weight gives shape to your muscles and makes you look fit.

Weight training will speed up your metabolism and will continue the fat burning process.

You can weight-train 3-5 days a week depending on your time availability. You should aim for 3 times a week minimum.

But first, you must learn all the exercises and practice in front of a mirror to make sure that you execute them right.

If this is your first-time using weights, just do whole body workouts, meaning one to two exercises per body part.

Once you get stronger and master the exercises you can work two body parts per work out and do a split based on how many workouts you will do er week.

Try to limit rest times to one minute or less between sets. This way, you keep the intensity of your workout high.

But if you feel that you need a bit longer to recover from an exercise then by all means do this.

Just don't take too long.

If you have already had experience with weights, then after giving yourself a couple of weeks to get back on track you can either increase the intensity or add a couple of more difficult exercises.

Another thing you can do to keep your intensity high to maintain the fat burning process is to do short HIIT workouts.

High Intensity Interval Training is short but intense burst of energy like jumps, of using light weights and doing an exercise for a certain amount of time-like 20-30 seconds.

Another way to increase the intensity and burn fat is doing exercise like jumping jacks or jump rope (with or without an actual rope) between the weight sets.

However, this is more advanced way, and you should give yourself some time to increase your fitness level before doing that.

Don't do this with every single workout though because you'll soon get tired, and you won't be able to keep up with the weight training.

In any case, see how your body feels before you go into deeper waters. This is not a competition; just a challenge to yourself.

How to organize your workouts

Here are sample routines you can use.

Here is one example of how to organize your training days and which muscle groups you can train together. It's not written in stone that you must do it this way, but it'll give you an idea of how you should group your training days.

Sample routine 1

4 days a week

<u>Monday</u>

Shoulders and biceps

<u>Tuesday</u>

Legs and abs

<u>Wednesday</u>

Only cardio

<u>Thursday</u>

Back and abs

<u>Friday</u>

Chest and triceps

Sample routine 2

4 days a week

<u>Monday</u>

Back and biceps

<u>Tuesday</u>

Chest and triceps

<u>Wednesday</u>

Legs and abs

<u>Thursday</u>

Cardio only

<u>Friday</u>

Shoulders and abs

Sample routine 3

5 days a week

<u>Monday</u>

Shoulders

<u>Tuesday</u>

Back

<u>Wednesday</u>

Legs

<u>Thursday</u>

Chest

<u>Friday</u>

Biceps and triceps

Note: You can do abs and cardio 4 days a week as well.

You can also train with weights three days a week if you prefer.

But this will mean a longer workout each day, and in the end you may tire more. Find the most convenient schedule for you.

This should be easy for you to follow so you don't get tempted to skip.

You should stick to the same routine for approximately two months. Give your body time to learn and adjust to the demands of the workout.

Don't be discouraged if you don't see results immediately. Have faith in the process and be persistent.

Don't ever give up. The results will come with repetition, focus, and determination.

And remember, now is the time to act. Don't let life pass you by. If you don't make a change today, you will end up like many women out there—frustrated, out of shape, and regretting that they never took action for themselves.

Being a good wife, mother, employee, and friend boils down to one thing: being satisfied with yourself first. Prioritizing everyone else's needs is certainly not the way to achieve that.

Of course, no two individuals are the same. A lot of the progress you'll make depends on your genetics, your status and weight, and any weaknesses that need your special attention.

Genetics is one thing, and working to overcome your weaknesses is another. Everyone can change physically. Your genetics may not predispose you to be a track and field champion, but you can dramatically improve your physique regardless.

My own family tends to be overweight. It's in our genes, but I chose early on not to let that dominate my life.

I've seen women and men in terrible physical condition who one day made the decision to change, escaping debilitating illness and early death. And they did it

Body shape

Your initial shape is important. Look at yourself in the mirror. Is your body more like a pear or an apple shape?

Most women have a pear shape, narrower upper body, and larger lower body. This means that they gain fat mostly around the hips and thighs.

The apple shaped body is the one that tends to put on weight around the belly and upper body. The lower body and legs are straight.

This natural body shape will tell you what body part you need to work on more.

For example, if you are pear-shaped, even after you lose all the weight, you will still have a smaller and weaker upper frame. As your training progresses, you might need to focus more on developing symmetry in the upper body.

If you are apple shaped, you may need to work more on shaping your legs. You are the one to decide that, depending on how satisfied you are with your progress.

Resistance variation and adaptation

When you first start training, go easy. Progressing too quickly by lifting too heavy too soon or overdoing your workouts will not accelerate your advancement.

For the initial couple of months, choose a resistance that allows you to complete approximately 12-15 repetitions for both the upper and lower body.

Once you get a grip on things, you can aim for a range of about 10-12 repetitions. Ensure you use the full range of motion, meaning you must fully extend and contract the muscle before moving into the next repetition.

This approach stimulates the entire muscle and yields optimal results. While many training techniques can fine-tune and sculpt a great physique, let's table that discussion for later.

Of course, you can't use the same resistance indefinitely. Over time, and as you progress, your muscles and strength will develop, becoming accustomed to the consistent resistance.

Your ability to do more without feeling fatigued will be a clear sign that you can increase your weight. The body possesses a remarkable ability to adapt to nearly any situation as part of our survival mechanism.

The same principle applies to cardio. Let's say you run on the treadmill every day for 20 minutes at a consistent speed. Initially, running the full 20 minutes may be challenging, but in time it will become substantially easier as your body adapts.

At this juncture, consider either extending the duration slightly or altering the exercise by increasing the incline and walking instead. When your body acclimates too thoroughly to your current workout, results may plateau.

If you frequent a gym, you can observe people who do the same unvarying routine every day and you can see they do not change at all.

The peril of comfort zones lies precisely in their comfort. This paradigm holds true in daily life as well. Consider those who vehemently dislike their jobs yet abstain from pursuing change, complaining persistently without ever submitting an application for a new position.

No one will spontaneously offer you a thrilling, well-compensated position, just as no one will modify your body for you. It is YOU who must pursue your desires.

Indeed, exiting your comfort zone demands effort and determination; superior job offers won't miraculously appear.

The same applies to fitness. To attain the body you want, to become fit, to enjoy robust health, to emulate a physique you admire, you must venture beyond your comfort zone and challenge yourself.

The importance of warming up

Warming up is not just for passing the time until you start with cardio or weights. It's an important part of your workout. It helps your body prepare for activity.

It prepares your muscles and heart for greater stress so you can train without injuring yourself. You can either warm up by doing 5-10 min of cardio or you can do it with very light weights.

Never start running on the treadmill or lifting weights without doing a couple of light warm up sets before.

If you sustain an injury, the healing process will typically be more protracted after the age of 40. Consequently, adopting a mindful approach to your workouts to minimize the risk of injury becomes paramount.

The exercises

Here are some exercises that are great to improve & develop different body parts.

Abdominals

Of course, you have heard of, seen, or done something called crunches. This exercise has several variations that you can try and rotate in your training—but only if you are not just starting out.

Crunches with feet positioned high at a 90° angle.

Twisting crunches

Reverse crunches

Stability ball crunches

Leg raises.

Side bend

Sit up.

Twisting sit up.

Incline sit up.

Chest

Bench press—flat or incline

Dumbbell fly

Dumbbell press

Pullover

Push up.

Shoulders

Lateral raises

Front raises

Seated dumbbell press

Alternating dumbbell press

Military press

Upright row

Bent over flys.

Back

Wide grip lateral pull down.

Reverse close grip lateral pull down.

Seated close grip lateral row.

Bent over barbell row.

One arm dumbbell bent over row.

T-bar row

Legs

Squats

Deadlift

Leg press

Front and back lunges

Walking lunges

Dead lift

Step up.

Cable kick back

Abductor machine

Leg extension

Lying leg curl

Biceps

Bicep curl

Hammer curl

Seated alternating curl.

Concentration curl

Barbell curl

Triceps

Press down with rope.

Triceps kickback

Dips

Behind the neck extension

Triceps extension

These are some of the best exercises you can do. Keep in mind, though, that to make a difference, you must practice the right form.

If an exercise is new to you, learn the proper form and start light before jumping into a strength building regime.

Don't ever forget to warm up before exercise and stretch afterwards. Take good care of your body and make sure you avoid injuries.

Key Body parts focus

Back

Having a strong back is not just about looking good. A healthy back becomes especially important as we age.

Having a healthy back will prevent problems that arise when you use weak muscles to lift groceries, do the housework, or sit at your desk for many hours every day.

Strong back muscles will keep your body upright and prevent lower back pain. They make your shoulders look wider, your abdominal area tighter, and your waist look smaller.

Train your back twice a week (after you go through with the initial beginning phase). Include exercises that work all three parts - **upper, middle, and lower** back - so that your muscles are equally strong.

For the best results, change exercises or repetitions for your second workout each week, or every four to six weeks.

The best back exercises are pulls, either seated or standing, with barbells or dumbbells or cables.

Shoulders

Your shoulder muscle is composed of three different heads: front, middle, and rear. All three need to be worked so that your shoulders have a fuller, rounded appearance.

Shoulders can be injured easily, so make sure to warm up well before you start your workout.

Exercises such as lateral raises, front raises, military presses, bent-over lateral raises, and pull-ups with a front barbell are among the best for building shoulder muscles.

Quads, hamstrings, and glutes.

Legs possess the largest muscles in the body, and it's necessary to work in all different areas, including the front, side, and back.

Nicely sculpted legs are a dream for women of all ages. They are also the first to be affected when you gain weight and fat.

Legs can quickly lose their shape when you don't exercise, particularly as we age and potentially adopt a more sedentary lifestyle, providing cellulite a place to settle.

The best exercises for achieving strong, sculpted legs include squats with a barbell or dumbbells, hip thrusts, leg presses, front, side, and back lunges, walking lunges, deadlifts, leg extensions, lying leg curls, and standing calf raises.

You can target your glutes or hamstrings with specific exercise combinations that focus more on those muscles. Doing these exercises will get you the best legs you've ever had.

There's no need to perform them all at once. Simply select four each time and rotate them to infuse variety into your training.

Sample exercise routines

Routine 1 (Upper Body)

Bench press

Incline dumbbell fly

Lateral raise

Dumbbell press

Triceps extension –w/cable

Bench dip

Sample routine 2 (Legs & Abs)

Dumbbell squat

Back lunges (alternate legs)

Lying leg curls

Standing calf raises

Crunches

Hanging leg raise-knee up

Sample routine 3 (Back, Biceps, Abs)

Wide grip pull down

Close grip pull down

Seated row-w/close grip

Bent over row.

Dumbbell curls-(alternate)

Barbell curls

Concentration curl

Crunches

Sample routine 4 (Full Body)

Incline bench dumbbell press

Incline fly

Seated bicep curls-(alternate)

Hummer curls

Barbell squats

Lying leg curl

Lateral raise

Front raise

Triceps press down.

Dips

Sample routine 1 (Legs)

Do a superset with the first two exercises, which means you perform one set of each exercise back-to-back without resting in between.

Rest after you finish both. (2 sets of 15 reps)

Barbell Squat

Back Lunges

Do 3 sets of 15 reps for each of the following exercises:

Deadlift

Leg extension

Kickback

Sample routine 2 (Legs)

Do a superset for the first 2 exercises. Rest after you finish both. (2 sets of 15 reps)

Leg press

Side lunge

Do 3 sets of 15 reps for each of the following exercises:

Hip thrusts.

Hamstrings curl

Walking lunges

Alternate these routines on your leg days.

Sample routine 1 (Shoulders)

Do 3 sets of 8 -10 repetitions for each exercise.

Front raises

Seated dumbbell press

Lateral raise

Incline side lateral raise

Sample routine 2(Shoulders)

Do 3 sets per exercise with 8-10 repetitions in each set.

Bent over fly.

Upright row

Lateral raise/ superset with

Front raise

Do only 2 sets for the last two exercises (superset).

Alternate these routines for two months and then increase the weight a bit.

Sample routine 1(Back)

Do 3 sets per exercise with 10-12 repetitions in each set.

Pull down front wide grip.

Pull down front close grip.

Seated row

One arm dumbbell row

Sample routine 2 (Back)

Do 3 sets per exercise with 8-10 repetitions in each set.

Bent over row.

Seated row

Machine pull up.

T-bar row

Alternate these routines when you work on your back. As you progress you can add more weight.

Sample routine 1 (Biceps and triceps)

Do 3 sets per exercise with 10-12 repetitions in each set.

Bicep curl

Bicep curl with barbell

Triceps press down.

Triceps kickbacks

Sample routine 2 (Bicep and triceps)

Do 3 sets per exercise with 10-12 repetitions in each set, and alternate routines on alternate arm days.

Barbell curl

Hammer cable curl

Seated dumbbell curl

Triceps overhead extension

Lying triceps extension

Dips with bench

*If you exercise at home and you don't have access to equipment/machine required for some of the exercises, simply leave those exercises out and replace them with another one that is easily done with dumbbells.

Circuit Training

Circuit training involves performing two or more exercises - usually between 3-5, with little or no rest between them, at a rather fast pace.

Circuits can be a lot of fun and they are very effective when it comes to cardiovascular conditioning and burning fat.

With circuits you can do any kind of jumps, sprints, or push-ups, or perform the same exercises you do when you weight train- only with much less weight.

Sample short circuit training workouts

Improve cardiovascular conditioning and burn fat.

Circuit 1

Do the following three exercises one after the other for 20 repetitions or 30 seconds. Then rest for one and a half minute and repeat the circuit 2 more times. Hold light weights.

Squats

Dead lift

Alternate front lunges with dumbbells

Circuit 2

Do the following three exercises one after the other for 20 repetitions or 30 seconds. Then rest for 1 minute and 30 seconds and repeat the circuit 2 more times. Hold light weights.

Alternate back lunge with bicep curl

Side lunge

Knee up hands overhead push

Circuit 3

Do the following three exercises one after the other for 20 repetitions or 30 seconds. Then rest for 1 minute and 30 seconds and repeat the circuit 2 more times. Use a Swiss ball.

Crunches on the ball

Legs up with the ball between the legs

Circuit 4

Do the following three exercises one after the other for 20 repetitions or 30 seconds. Then rest for 1 minute and 30 seconds and repeat the circuit 2 more times.

Back extension on the ball

Push up either on your knees or regular. Try to do as many as you can. This is a difficult exercise, and you need to build up your strength.

Circuit trainings can be integrated into any of your workouts or just do them separately when you are short of time.

Circuits are great for burning fat, and they also sculpt and define your muscles.

Because they require endurance, you might not be able to do the whole circuit at the beginning.

Try to complete 10 repetitions of the first exercise and then move on to the next for another 10.

Rest and try again.

You will eventually work your way up to finishing the whole circuit.

Try to integrate circuits training into your routine at least once or twice a week.

Circuits can also be done in your yard, at home, or even at the park.

You'll soon witness a remarkable transformation in your physique. While these are mere examples, feel free to create your own circuits as your fitness level advances.

Endless options exist. Yet, bear in mind that transformation requires effort. Nutrition is crucial, accounting for more than 70% of your success. Even with optimal gym practices, maintaining an unhealthy diet and consuming more than you burn will kill your efforts.

The journal

What to write in your journal?

Draw a matrix for your exercises. Include a space for the day of the week and the date. Then enter the body part you are working on, every exercise you do, the weight you used for each set, and repetitions accomplished.

Make sure to write down every set and every exercise. Also note how much time you spend on cardio activities and warming up.

Here is an example:

Monday, November 3rd

<u>Warm up</u>

10minuteson the bike

<u>Exercise weight/repetition:</u>

<u>Legs</u>

Lunges 8x208x2010x15

Leg extensions10x2010x2012x15

Squats10x1510x1510x15

<u>Abs</u>

Crunches 3x25

Knee up3x15

You get the idea. This will help you keep track of everything that you do and give you a way to measure progress.

Keep the same kind of record for your nutrition, right down the time and everything that you eat.

For example:

10.00 AM - Tuna sandwich with multigrain bread. - 1 apple.

1:00 PM - 1 grilled chicken breast

1 small green salad

1 small, sweet potato

1 cup low fat yogurt

1 cup coffee

Document any cravings and the specific foods you desire. It's vital to note instances of emotional or boredom-driven eating, such as late-night snacking in front of the TV. To address these issues, you must first identify them.

Supplements

Do you need any?

Every woman over 40 aiming to lose weight and engaging in physical activity should consider a quality multivitamin supplement.

Our nutrient requirements heighten with age, and our bodies may not absorb nutrients as efficiently as they once did. Additionally, the nutritional quality of many foods may not be as robust as it was two or three decades ago, given the prevalent use of pesticides and environmental toxins, which can saturate fruits and vegetables with chemicals rather than vitamins.

Studies indicate that consuming about five oranges a day is needed to meet the RDA (recommended daily allowance) of vitamin C. If that's achievable, you might forgo multivitamin supplements.

However, if, like me, you find it challenging to consume the necessary foods to meet your daily vitamin and mineral needs, opting for a multivitamin pill as a safety net is prudent.

I recommend that you take a **glucosamine-chondroitin** supplement.

Glucosamine helps your joints remain in good condition. It promotes cartilage formation and elasticity of the joint. Even if you don't experience or have any joint problems it's a good idea to start protecting them early.

L –Carnitin

L-Carnitin will help your body lose more fat. L-Carnitin is an amino acid involved in metabolism. It transports fatty acids through the body, so they convert into energy.

It will increase your metabolism and improve recovery time. This is important for women our age, as we tend to get tired more easily than before. We sure can use all the energy we can get.

Another great supplement is an **Omega-3** capsule. Better yet, consider taking a combination of omega-3 and omega-6.

They are both essential fatty acids that have been found to be extremely beneficial to general, and especially cardiovascular, health.

Omega 3 and 6 diminish inflammation of the veins, inhibit plaque formation in the arteries, and help protect against cancers like colon and breast cancer.

They also protect against inflammatory diseases like rheumatoid arthritis. So, if you live in a cold, humid climate this is something to consider.

I also recommend that you take **Berberin**, a natural supplement that helps with glucose metabolism. Women over 40 and beyond often have difficulty losing weight because of insulin resistance.

Turmeric is another great supplement that is a natural anti-inflammatory and prevents free radical and toxins damage.

Protein shakes

Should you drink any protein shakes?

Since you want to lose fat and support lean muscle tissue, I suggest that you take a good protein supplement.

Protein supplements come in powder or bars. Powder is what you should be looking for.

Nowadays, nutritional companies have made huge progress. The taste and composition of the proteins is amazing.

You can mix them with water or skim milk of yogurt for a delicious drink in between meals or whenever you feel hungry and can't access healthy food.

Protein shakes are good. They are convenient, easy to prepare, and a good way to get that all-important protein.

Now there are thousands of protein powders on the market.

Most of them are good but when you look for a good protein product, it's important to check out two things:

The first is the amount of protein per serving. It should be over 20gr. More is even better; and

The second is that you should be careful about the amount of carbohydrates.

Some of the proteins out there contain a very high percentage of carbohydrates, which tend to come from sugars.

Be careful what you buy. Have a good look at the ingredients list. Examine the carbohydrate content and select a brand with lower carbs.

Maintain a stash of protein bars with you, whether traveling or in the office, to mitigate temptations towards cakes and cookies.

Protein bars deliver the advantages of protein and offer convenient portability and consumption, even at work. However, many contain a significant amount of sugar, so consume them judiciously.

Protein, available in shakes, bars, or food, assists in preserving and potentially increasing muscle mass during fat loss.

Gut Health

Have you noticed that you feel like your digestion is off track? Do you feel as if everything you eat makes you feel like you've swallowed stones? If yes, your intestines and digestive system are not working properly.

Indigestive Issues

As time goes by, our digestive system loses its optimal function. There are plenty of reasons for that. One of them is that when you've eaten poorly for years, and have neglected proper and healthy nutrition, your digestive system becomes overloaded.

It works extra hard to digest high-fat, high-carb, highly processed, low-fiber foods and alcoholic drinks, which results in many of the foods you eat leaving an undesirable residue inside your intestines.

Often, this is also the cause of bloating, gas, and feeling very full and uncomfortable in your own skin. You also gain weight much faster and have difficulty losing it.

The positive news is that you can change this by altering your eating habits and adopting a healthier lifestyle.

Why detoxing your digestive system is vital?

Optimal health begins in the gut! If you've spent years overindulging in sugars, processed foods, chemicals, and abundant red meat while skimping on fiber and antioxidants, the repercussions may be becoming apparent as you approach 40.

You might already be experiencing food sensitivities and intolerances, all stemming from a longstanding, unhealthy diet.

To enhance gut health, improve digestion, and facilitate weight loss, it's crucial to acknowledge that a dietary shift is imperative.

Embarking on a diet rich in fiber and vegetables is a promising start. Additionally, incorporating a high-quality probiotic into your supplement routine and indulging in fermented foods like kimchi, kombucha (a type of fungus), and kefir is advisable.

These foods are laden with probiotics that encourage healthy gut bacteria and rejuvenate intestinal flora.

By revitalizing your gut health, you'll not only experience physical and mental enhancements, but you'll also notice a surge in energy, a reduction in stress, and an almost immediate beginning of weight loss.

Tips and tricks to help you lose weight.

Apple Cider Vinegar

Apple cider vinegar, a natural product with a long history of versatile uses, boasts numerous healing properties. It is commonly utilized to support healthy digestion, manage insulin sensitivity, and facilitate weight loss.

The theory behind this is that apple cider vinegar increases the acidity in the stomach and makes it easier to digest foods. You should be taking 1-2 spoons before a meal in an empty stomach (diluted in half glass of water).

You will also lose weight because apple cider vinegar gives you a sense of fullness and reduces appetite.

I've witnessed numerous clients achieve impressive results by complementing a healthy diet with apple cider vinegar. If you've been consuming high-carb meals and noticing a climb in your scale numbers, it's possible that you've developed insulin sensitivity unknowingly.

As highlighted earlier, dietary alterations are pivotal for improvement, but integrating apple cider vinegar can thwart sugar spikes post meals.

Consider trying intermittent fasting once a week. If you are new to the concept, intermittent fasting involves an eating pattern that alternates between eating and fasting periods, serving as a method to restrict calories and detox your body.

There are various approaches, but a beginner-friendly method is either 14/10 or 16/8, signifying 14 or 16 hours of fasting and eating during the remaining 10 or 8 hours.

If, for instance, your last meal is at 8 pm, and you wake up at 7 am, your first meal should be at 10 am or noon. During fasting, you may drink black coffee, unsweetened tea, and water.

This is your fasting window from 8 pm to 10 am for a 14/10 split. You can enjoy breakfast items like fruit, a protein shake, or cereal at your first meal, followed by lunch around 3 pm, and dinner around 8 pm, abstaining from eating after this but permitting beverages like coffee and tea.

Thus, you still consume three meals.

The 16/8 method simply shifts your first meal to noon and your last to 8 pm. This method provides flexibility as long as fasting times are adhered to and may be more conveniently implemented during weekends when social and dining-out activities are more common.

Engaging in a one-day-per-week fast carries several benefits. Firstly, managing hunger for just one day is typically more feasible. Conducting it over a weekend can be simpler because potentially sleeping in contributes to your fasting period, hastening the time until you can eat.

Although I generally advocate for the regular consumption of smaller meals and snacks, occasional fasting presents some advantages.

Primarily, you consume notably fewer calories, aiding in weight loss or maintenance while still enjoying a social dinner. It also mitigates insulin sensitivity and can stabilize blood sugar levels.

Lower insulin levels mean reduced fat storage susceptibility. Intermittent fasting can activate fat burning in the body.

Employing it once a week may recalibrate the body's internal clock, initiate an auto-cleansing process, and trigger Autophagy, where cells dispose of old, damaged proteins that accumulate inside them, potentially reducing inflammation which can lead to weight gain, hormonal imbalances, and other health issues.

Nevertheless, to realize these health benefits, you must adhere to consuming healthy foods and ample water during your eating window.

I must note, however, that I'm not a strong advocate of intermittent fasting as a perpetual eating pattern, since it can incite insatiable hunger, resulting in binge-eating and potential muscle mass loss if extended over long periods.

While it might seem clichéd, it's absolutely true: never skip breakfast. Breakfast is pivotal, breaking your body's eight-hour overnight fast and replenishing its fuel.

Departing without breakfast often leads to significant hunger shortly, thereafter, prompting people to overeat during subsequent meals and gravitate towards less healthy options, culminating in weight gain.

Maintain discipline with your schedule. Record your planned workouts in your calendar and honor the time reserved for them.

Post-exercise, you'll invariably feel better, and consistent repetition fosters habit development.

Abandon the phrase "I am on a diet." This is not a temporary diet; it's a lifestyle adjustment. You are not on a diet!

I have already pointed out that diets don't work, and that if you don't do things differently you will always get the same old results as before.

You are just reeducating yourself to eat differently.

Eat three meals and two snacks a day.

Eating often and in small quantities will speed up your metabolism and will help you lose weight.

Eat fruit with your breakfast instead of drinking juice.

In addition to vitamins, fruit contains fibers that make them digest slower.

This gives you the feeling of satiety. You have more energy, and you are not hungry.

Juices, on the other hand, go right through your body.

They get digested quickly and your blood sugar will rise and drop quickly.

This causes those cravings that make you end up eating more sweet things.

Try to eat a salad one hour before your dinner.

By starting with a fresh salad an hour or two before your main dish, you will cut your appetite at least by half.

Green or fresh fruit salads are very healthy and create a feeling of fullness.

By the time you sit down for dinner you won't even think of second servings or dessert.

You may not even finish what is on your plate.

Your appetite is under control and so is the amount of food you consume.

The leftover syndrome: if you have the habit of eating the last bits of food as you pick up your family's plates, you'll have to change this habit.

You either must throw the food in the garbage right after you pick up the plates or put it in a container and store it in the fridge for another day.

Leftovers are one of the main factors contributing to women's obesity. Don't fall into that trap.

Right after you finish working out, <u>drink a protein shake</u>.

Protein will help your muscles recuperate and grow, while it diminishes your appetite. Then have a meal 2-3 hours later.

Focus on complex carbohydrates and keep simple ones to a strict minimum.

All kinds of vegetables, like green beans, broccoli, peas, carrots, zucchini; and grains like lentils, brown rice, and chickpeas; are very good choices. If you must have pasta, it's better to have it at lunchtime than at dinner.

Limit alcohol consumption to weekends only. Or you can quit altogether.

Alcohol provides 7 calories per gram and is metabolized in the body as fat.

Drinking alcohol gives you many unnecessary calories and if you drink a lot, you will end up gaining weight.

If you must drink alcohol, choose dry wine.

Dry wine has antioxidants, does not contain extra sugar, and has a low alcohol content.

A glass or two during the weekend will do you good but remember not to exceed that amount.

Prepare all the snacks you need to take with you in advance. Prepare veggies like celery sticks, baby carrots, and peppers.

They will fill you up and are also very rich in vitamins and fiber.

You can also stock your desk at work with grains like almonds and walnuts in case you get hungry and can't go for lunch.

Always carry some protein powder to make a shake.

Plan your shopping before you go shopping. Make a quick list of what you will need to prepare your meals. If you are not exactly sure what to get, then chicken, turkey, and lean steak are always good choices.

You can always modify your recipes to make them healthier.

It's easy to cut the fat content in half. For example, instead of deep frying your meat and chicken, cook it in a skillet and drain the fat after cooking.

Diminish the number of whole eggs you eat per week. Limit them to three. You can make excellent omelets with egg whites that are 100% protein.

Buy low fat and nonfat milk and yogurt. Be careful with full fat dairy since it's loaded with saturated fat.

Other foods high in saturated fat include cheese, cream cheese, salami, cookies and pastries, butter, coconut and palm oil, and candies just to name a few. Avoid them.

These foods will not only make you gain weight, but they are bad for your health. They will raise your bad cholesterol and over time clog your arteries.

Since at our age we are more sensitive to the things we eat and drink, you must be aware of what you are doing to your health. Remember that your current body illustrates your eating habits and the state of your health.

Stop using sugar in your coffee or tea. Sugar adds a lot of extra calories that you can easily spare. You can use agave as a natural sweetener or another sugar substitute if you really can't have your coffee without a sweetener of some sort. You will have to use artificial sweetener with caution as they can create gut inflammation and bloating.

If you like coffee, try to stick to black or with low fat cream. Now there are many light creamers on the market but always check the label for the amount of sugar they contain.

You should completely forget about the tall latte with whip cream and other extras that you find at many coffee shops. These coffee drinks are calorie bombs. They contain between 600 to over 1000 calories! Yes, you read that right.

Put enough of those extras in your coffee and you'll end up with more calories than you get from a regular meal. In fact, depending on how many of these you add to your coffee you can finally get over half your daily calorie requirements just by drinking coffee.

Not to mention all the sugar and saturated fat you'll ingest.

By making small changes and reeducating yourself regarding food choices, you will take huge steps towards achieving your weight loss goal and attaining the body you've always wanted, even after the age of forty.

If you just do some simple math, you'll soon realize that every time you take a second serving it adds up to about 150/200 extra calories.

If you have seconded a few times a week - if not every day - calculate how many calories, you add weekly to your body.

All these extra calories lead to a steady weight gain each year.

Then when the hard reality hits and you have 20, 30 or more pounds to lose, it isn't going to be easy.

As we get older, we need to take care of our bodies even more than when we were 25 or 30.

It's not just a question of how we look. Remember that with extra weight, health problems appear as well.

Back problems and knee problems are the most common ones.

If you don't train your muscles, your skin will start to loosen and become flabby around your arms, belly, and thighs.

You'll start looking older than your real age. Your self-confidence will drop and people around you will sense it.

We live in a very competitive society and if you want to enjoy the job that you love so much it's important to keep in shape.

I know there are many different opinions out there, but weight discrimination is real and is not going to disappear any time soon whether you accept it or not.

The same goes for your marriage or relationship. You might think your partner will always love you no matter your looks but when your weight climbs up it might become an issue.

And this goes both ways. I have worked with many ladies that their relationships have suffered ever since they started putting on weight.

Building up the body that you want will give you confidence, strength of character, persistence, and discipline.

This is a wonderful journey, and you will enjoy it.

The cellulite curse.

What is cellulite - Why do you have it - What to do about it?

As you may know, 'cellulite' refers to the unsightly dimples arising from localized fat forming beneath the skin. At various points in life, most women, regardless of age, grapple with cellulite.

Numerous factors contribute to the development of cellulite, including hormonal shifts, poor diet, a sedentary lifestyle, weight gain, and pregnancy. The quest to eradicate cellulite has been an ongoing battle for years.

Many women, confronted with this persistent issue, decide to accept it as it is. When weight is gained, these troublesome and unsightly dimples often make their appearance around the hips and belly.

Additionally, they may manifest on the backs of arms, particularly where the skin has lost its tightness, possibly due to a lack of exercise. While men also experience cellulite, women tend to encounter it more frequently.

Furthermore, most men are not as perturbed by its presence to actively seek its removal.

3 Stages of Cellulite

Believe it or not, cellulite has 3 different stages.

Stage 1 is the hard cellulite, the lightest. This type is more common in young adolescents or older women. It becomes visible when your muscles are relaxed, and you squeeze the skin firmly with both hands.

Stage 2 is the so-called "orange peel." In this stage we can see cellulite regardless of whether the person is standing or sitting. The skin develops ugly dimples and by squeezing we can feel the hard spots under the skin.

Stage 3 is the advanced stage of cellulite. Here we can see holes in the surface of the skin and squeezing it is painful.

Although the initial stage of cellulite is often nearly invisible, the subsequent two stages involve its stabilization, during which blood and lymph circulation becomes disrupted, potentially making edemas visible. In these advanced stages, alterations in nutrition and daily exercise are imperative to observe improvements.

As we age, cellulite tends to become more apparent and increasingly challenging to eliminate. Several factors contribute to this.

One such factor is years of fat storage, coupled with a lack of exercise and poor eating habits. Such a lifestyle exacerbates cellulite, and to mitigate it, a shift in eating habits is crucial. It's advisable to avoid foods like sweets, cakes, snacks, potato chips, lunch meats, ready-to-eat foods, café lattes, and whipped cream, to name a few.

Another catalyst for cellulite development is the hormonal changes occurring throughout a woman's life. It's noteworthy that cellulite can affect even very young women and is not exclusively tied to age.

However, if you are utilizing birth control pills or taking hormones for other reasons, you might be more susceptible to developing cellulite, since contraceptive pills maintain higher hormone levels in your body to prevent pregnancy.

Since hormones circulate in your body without asking your permission, there isn't much you can do about it.

Before menstruation or menopause, your hormone levels might rise or fall dramatically. These changes in hormones are responsible for the bloated feeling you might have and for the cellulite around your belly and thighs.

In that case, topical lotions and creams can improve the quality of your skin. Regular exercise is a must, in combination with nutritional changes. It also helps if you drink a lot of water.

There are natural ways to balance your hormones and indirectly easy the appearance of cellulite.

Another reason for having cellulite is water retention.

If you have a medical condition or simply eat a lot of high sodium foods, water retention is a factor that contributes to cellulite. Drinking a lot of good quality water helps with the elimination process.

You can add mild, natural diuretics like herbal teas to your daily routine. They help with cellulite and release any pressure associated with water retention.

Again, nutritional changes are necessary. Exercise is particularly recommended in this case.

Bad nutrition is a major culprit.

If fast food restaurants, high fat snacks, alcohol, and sodas are your first choice when it comes to food, stop. People who eat a lot of carbohydrates (more than they need), and a lot of salt, usually have apparent cellulite.

Frequent alcohol use contributes, as well. If you have at least one drink every day, then you probably will have to reduce your consumption to reduce your cellulite.

A sedentary lifestyle is another main reason for developing cellulite. If you get little to no exercise and you spend most of the day behind your desk, you are creating a positive environment for cellulite to settle in. You need to activate your blood circulation, build up some muscle, and tone your whole body to combat cellulite.

Other causes of cellulite include smoking, stress, and post-partum weight accumulation.

In every single case of cellulite, you must consider nutritional changes.

I cannot stress this enough.

Drink a lot of water, at least one liter or ½ gallon per day. I recommend that you have a few glasses per day diluted with fresh lemon juice.

Lemon has detoxifying qualities and will help your body get rid of toxins that cause cellulite.

It is also an excellent antioxidant, will help your digestion, and is abundant in vitamin C.

Here are a few additional foods that can aid in combating cellulite: grapefruit, pineapple, and asparagus, all of which are excellent for those experiencing water retention.

If you have the budget for salon treatments, massages help improve circulation and mobilize fat cells for excretion. Wrapping is one of the best treatments for cellulite.

It must be done by a professional beautician and involves applying an anti-cellulite crème to the lower body or other affected parts, and then wrapping you up in a sort of strong plastic wrap.

This helps your body get rid of toxins and makes your skin look amazingly improved after a session.

You must get the treatment on a regular basis to maintain results.

Another great procedure is endermology.

A professional massage therapist operates a little machine that rolls slowly over your affected parts. You put on a special legging, and the machine simply sucks and rolls your skin.

It helps break down stubborn fat deposits and mobilizes them for excretion from the body. You will have to drink plenty of water to facilitate the excretion process.

Endermology is rather expensive, and it takes at least 10 sessions of for results to become visible.

But, if you can afford it, I recommend checking it out.

Remember to regularly exfoliate your body and apply a good anti-cellulite cream to affected body parts afterwards.

Another good trick is to use a bath glove to massage your legs and thighs, starting from low to high. You can start from your ankles doing slow circular moves all the way up to hips and inner thighs.

This is a simple action but very effective because it activates blood circulation in the area and moves the accumulated toxins all the way up to the lymph nodes to be excreted from the body.

This will tremendously improve the appearance of your skin, and it maintains anti-cellulite-action. After every massage session you should always apply a firming anti-cellulite crème.

Another simple yet effective thing you can do, especially during the winter months, is to buy and wear compression pantyhose. These are usually for women suffering from varicose veins and look exactly like the regular ones.

They are specially designed to press and massage the leg from your ankle all the way up. You can usually find them at your pharmacy or ask your pharmacist to order it for you.

Remember that this is a long process so never give up.

Navigating Social Events on Your Wellness Journey

Social events, whether they are work-related or family gatherings, invariably center around food and drink and are an inevitable aspect of life.

Striking a balance between participating in these events and adhering to your weight loss goals can undoubtedly pose a challenge.

You might find yourself fielding questions or being met with a lack of understanding, or even dealing with potentially offended hosts or guests when you refrain from indulging in certain foods and beverages.

To circumvent the stress and sidestep the need for lengthy explanations about your dietary choices, being prepared is key.

Let's explore some strategies to employ the next time you find an invitation to a party or barbecue in your inbox.

#1 Prepare in advance.

Before you leave your house, have a meal that's preferably high in protein and veggies.

For example, you can have some cottage cheese with cherry tomatoes. This will keep you full, and you won't be hungry and will start eating everything you find in the kitchen cabinets without consideration.

#2 At the party, use smaller dishes and don't stuff your plate with food. Just put few things on and eat slowly while you stay social and engage in conversations with people.

Remind yourself that the reason you are there is not to get a free giant meal, that's not going to do you any favors when it comes to weight loss.

This will distract you from food.

#3 Drink plenty of water the entire day.

You will be hydrated have less appetite and you won't feel so tempted to try everything that's available.

Remember: Food at events or family reunions is not made with your weight loss goals in mind.

#4 Be careful with alcohol.

If you decide to have a drink, get something lighter like wine spritzers or light beers. The better option will be to have a light soda with ice so people will not really know what you drink, and you can always say that you have some sort of cocktail.

Remember, alcohol contains empty calories -that have no nutritional value- and can increase your appetite for poorer food choices.

#5 Try to stay active as much as you can.

For example, you can help the host clean the dishes, or tide up, you can dance, or walk around the garden if that's a possibility.

#6 Make smart choices:

Once you see what's available decide to eat the healthier choices like grilled vegetables or lean meats and salads.

Just avoid fried and greasy foods, everything that has creamy sauces or sugary desserts.

#7 Make smart beverage choices:

If you decide not to drink alcohol that's great.

But the absence of alcohol doesn't mean the beverage is a great choice. It's not just alcoholic beverages that can sabotage your weight loss.

High sugary juices and syrups are really, really something you should avoid. Choose instead unsweetened tea, black coffee, tomato juice or a glass of sparkling water infused with fresh fruits or herbs.

#8 The uncomfortable situation eating:

Don't eat just to compensate for feeling awkward. Surely there were times where you have you been invited somewhere but you realized that you don't feel at ease.

I'm sure you have tried to deal with this by drinking or eating just to avoid talking to people or to make yourself feel comfortable.

If you find yourself in this kind of situation don't try to make yourself, feel better by eating or drinking mindlessly.

Instead focus on applying all the strategies mentioned here and try to shorten your stay as much as you can.

Your road map.

As I've said repeatedly above, I'm against dieting and diets. I simply don't believe that they ever help anybody. Diets only contribute to people's weight problems.

Women spend so much of their adult lives on diets, but they never learn how to keep the weight off. If diets were the right way to lose weight and keep it off, then every single woman out there would be thin today.

I just tell my clients that eating right is the only right way. To lose the weight and keep it off you must pay attention to the following points:

1. Exercise.

I can't stress enough the importance of including exercise in your daily routine. No matter how old or how young you are, you must exercise.

This is one of the best time investments you will ever make. Don't fool yourself into thinking that you can change without having to exercise.

Pay attention to how much food you eat.

We tend to underestimate the quantity of food we are putting onto our plates and into our bodies.

Learn to estimate the right portion size.

2. Be consistent.

Once you make the decision to achieve the best body of your life, don't look back. Follow correct eating habits not only on weekdays but also on the weekends.

Try not to spoil a good effort by eating like there is not tomorrow.

3. Always eat breakfast before you leave home

Fuel your body at the right time and program yourself for success. Don't skip meals and do everything you can to eat at regular intervals of 3 to 4 hours.

4. Control your weight once a week

I know that at the beginning you may be scared to look at the number on the scale, but you need to get used to recording your progress.

Weight control should become a habit. You should be able to see a difference in the way your clothes fit. But be careful - although you need to check your weight once a week, you don't need to become obsessed with the number on the scale.

The number you see on the scale may be going down slowly but the most important thing is to lose fat. Do what you need to do, and the results will come.

5. Emphasizing the importance of getting enough sleep

Adequate sleep each night is paramount not only for rest but also for bodily regeneration. To maintain a vibrant appearance and feel your best, it's wise to avoid late-night TV binges, extended partying, or any activities that could shorten your sleep.

Surprisingly, insufficient sleep can also contribute to weight gain. Indeed, various studies indicate that a lack of sufficient sleep can trigger a hormonal imbalance, complicating weight loss efforts.

When sleep evades you, hunger often kicks in, tempting midnight snacking when you should be resting. Your body demands more calories to sustain its additional awake time, making late-night eating a risky business.

Once you begin eating late at night, stopping can be a struggle. While satisfying initial hunger pangs, the solitude of nightfall, free from judgmental eyes, might entice you to continue eating until nothing remains.

Even if you resist the urge to raid the fridge, your body might interpret your wakefulness as a need to conserve energy, thereby holding onto its reserves.

However, consistently adhering to your exercise routine typically results in pleasant fatigue by day's end, promoting a deep, restful sleep. You'll likely awaken feeling refreshed and eager to start your day with a nutritious breakfast.

Compose your own meal plan.

Here are examples of different meals and snacks you can choose from. You can mix them and make your eating plan, or you can adjust according to your likes and dislikes.

Just make sure you replace them with foods that you can have and not with the ones that you should avoid.

Breakfasts

Sample 1

Omelet, with 4 egg whites and 1 whole egg

2 slices turkey ham

2 Tablespoons low fat cottage cheese

1 slice whole wheat multi grain bread

Coffee or tea with no sweeteners

Sample 2

2 cups cooked oatmeal

½ cup blueberries or strawberries

1 cup skim milk or soy milk

Coffee or tea with no sweeteners

Sample 3

1 slice whole wheat or multi grain bread with

1 Tablespoon natural peanut butter or natural almond butter.

1 kiwi, or 1 apple, or ½ cup blueberries

1 cup natural low-fat yogurt

Coffee or tea with no sweeteners

Sample 4

1 low fat turkey sausage

2 Tablespoons low fat cottage cheese

1 slice multi grain bread

1 apple

Coffee or tea with no sweeteners

Lunch

Sample 1

Chicken breast grilled with

Chopped tomato and cucumber.

1 cup brown rice

Use olive oil on the tomato and cucumber or a fat free dressing.

Sample 2

Green salad with tuna fish canned in water.

Add 1 Tablespoon of low-fat cottage cheese.

1 chopped tomato.

3 natural walnuts, chopped.

Add fresh lemon juice and 1 teaspoon of olive oil.

1 apple or orange

Sample 3

1 bowl lentil soup

1 slice whole grain bread

2 slices turkey ham

1 apple or orange

Sample 4

Sandwich with whole grain bread

Canned chicken breast in water mixed with 2-4 spoon full of low-fat cottage cheese and chopped pepper and onions. Add fresh lemon juice or a half teaspoon of olive oil, depending on consistency.

1 small bowl fresh fruit salad (Use only chopped fresh fruits, not canned).

Dinner

Sample 1

Grilled salmon or other kind of fish with

1 cup brown rice

1 cup green beans steamed or boiled.

1 Tablespoon of olive oil and lemon juice on the vegetables

Sample 2

Sirloin steak grilled with

½ sweet potato, baked

1 cup mixed vegetables, broccoli, cauliflower, and carrots steamed or boiled with a Tablespoon of olive oil.

Sample 3

2 medium size tortillas filled with tomato sauce, grilled chicken or turkey breast diced, green and yellow peppers sliced, and 2 Tablespoons grated low fat cheese.

1 small bowl of green salad with 1 Tablespoon olive oil.

1 cup low fat yogurt

Sample 4

Minced turkey meat grilled with

2 cups spinach and bulgur mixed.

½ sweet potato boiled

1 small bowl fruit salad mixed. (Only fresh seasonal fruits - no cans).

Snacks

As I have mentioned in previous chapters, having protein shakes as snacks and after your workout will make you feel full, keep your metabolic rate high, and start the fat loss process.

Here are some good options for you.

Sample 1

1 cup low fat yogurt

4 natural walnuts

Sample 2

1 rice cake with

1 slice turkey ham

1 egg white boiled

Sample 3

Carrots and celery sticks with

½ cup low fat cottage cheese

Sample 4

1 whole wheat cracker with

1 Tablespoons natural peanut butter

Section 2

Healthy Recipes

Dive into these recipes as you embark on your journey to transform your body. Not only do they offer a variety of flavors, but, when paired with your exercise regimen, they'll also assist you in shedding fat and building muscle

Spicy chicken

6 ounces chicken breast cut in chunks.

1 can diced tomatoes, or 2 fresh tomatoes diced.

1 can spicy hot chili beans

1 medium onion chopped.

Sauté the chicken breast and onions in a pan with a bit of olive oil. Stir in the tomatoes and beans. Cook for 10 minutes Sprinkle with low fat cheddar cheese (optional).

Fajitas

1 oz lean red meat cut in small pieces.

1 large green pepper cut into strips.

1 red pepper cut in strips.

1 medium yellow onion cut into strips.

Garlic for flavor

1 Tablespoon chili powder

Lemon juice

Fresh pepper

Use a large skillet or wok to sauté the garlic with lemon juice. Add the meat and the chili powder and cook until the meat is done to the degree you prefer.

Add the peppers and onions and cook until the vegetables are soft. Put the whole mixture into a whole wheat tortilla and top with salsa.

Chicken Cacciatore

2 lbs boneless and skinless chicken breast

1 can crushed tomato.

1 chopped onion

1 chopped green pepper.

1 pressed garlic clove

¼ Tablespoon thyme

½ Tablespoon parsley

½ Tablespoon oregano

Dash of pepper

½ Tablespoon Salt

Cooking spray

Spray pan with cooking spray and heat. Brown chicken and set aside.

Add chopped onion, green pepper, and garlic. Cook for about 5 minutes, then add the crushed tomatoes, parsley, oregano, salt, and pepper.

Cook on low for about 15 minutes, stirring occasionally, then add the chicken and cook for about 45 min on low.

Uncover and cook for 10 additional minutes. Serve with brown rice.

Pan broiled fish.

1 lbs fish fillets

1 14 oz can dice tomatoes with basil, garlic, and oregano.

Arrange the fish fillets in a single layer in a skillet.

Cover with tomatoes and liquid; add garlic, salt, and oregano.

Cook on medium heat for about 20 minutes. Serve with brown rice or cooked sweet potato.

Broiled fish Dijon

6 fish fillets

1 ½ lbs small zucchini, cut lengthwise in halves.

½ cup lemon juice

2 Tablespoons Dijon mustard

1 clove garlic minced.

2 Tablespoons drained capers

Paprika for taste

Rinse fish and pat dry. In a separate bowl stir together mustard and garlic.

Arrange fish and zucchini in a single layer in a large pan and drizzle lemon juice over it. Broil on the top rack for 5 minutes. Turn the fish over and spread with mustard and garlic mixture. Continue to broil for 5 minutes or until the zucchini is lightly browned and the fish cooked.

Sprinkle with paprika and capers.

Stuffed chicken breasts

1 chopped onion

1 pack frozen spinach thawed and dried.

1 egg lightly beaten.

8 oz low fat ricotta cheese

Salt and pepper

4 boneless, skinless chicken breasts, sliced in half and flattened.

Combine the onion, spinach, egg, and cheese in a bowl and mix.

Put a dollop of the mixture into each chicken breast.

Tie the chicken breasts together with butcher's twine or put toothpicks through them.

Bake at 350 degrees for 30-35 minutes.

Ground turkey breast with sauce

1lb ground turkey or beef

1 chopped onion

1 cup chopped portabella mushrooms.

1 Tablespoon red pepper flakes

1 teaspoon allspice

Salt and pepper

1 jar spaghetti sauce

Brown the meat with the red pepper flakes. Add the chopped onion and mushrooms. Add the allspice, salt, and pepper. Pour in the spaghetti sauce. Serve with brown rice, couscous, or yam.

Grilled chicken asparagus rolls

1 chicken breast

2 asparagus sticks

2 slices of low-fat turkey bacon

1 Tablespoon Dijon mustard

Salt and pepper

Cut the skinless chicken breast into slices and cover them with salt, pepper, and mustard.

Let marinate for 25 minutes.

Wash and peel the asparagus, then place a slice of bacon on each side of the chicken breast.

Place one asparagus stick on the top and start rolling it.

Use toothpicks to secure the bacon and make sure you place them in such a way that the chicken maintains its shape around the roll. You can grill or bake the rolls until meat is done.

Garlic roasted vegetables.

6 carrots peeled and quartered.

6 parsnips peeled and quartered.

6 shallots peeled and halved.

2 medium onions peeled and cut into 6-8 wedges.

1 large garlic bulb, broken into cloves and peeled.

1 Tablespoon dried thyme

4 Tablespoons olive oil

Preheat oven to 400 degrees.

Combine all the vegetables in a roasting pan, drizzle with oil and stir to coat.

Roast for about one hour and 20 minutes until they are tender.

You can also use the grill. Combine all the vegetables in a tinfoil bag, drizzle with olive oil, and stir. Roast for about 30 minutes until they are tender.

Combine it with meat, chicken, or fish.

Fish in foil

½ lbs halibut cut in two pieces

1 tomato chopped.

1 green onion chopped.

4 small zucchinis, julienned

1 cup dry white wine

1 Tablespoon each fresh dill and parsley

Dash of fresh ground pepper

Preheat oven to 400 degrees.

Cut two 12-inch square pieces of foil. Place a piece of fish on each square of foil.

Top each piece of fish with tomato, green onion, zucchini, and carrot.

Sprinkle each with wine, herbs, and pepper. Fold foil edges together, sealing with a pleat. Bake for 15 minutes.

Protein smoothie

1 cup fat free milk

1 cup fat free vanilla yogurt

1/3 cup frozen blueberries

¼ cup eggbeaters

½ banana

Toss all the ingredients together into a blender and blend until smooth.

Protein pancakes

6 egg whites

1 cup oats

2 scoops whey protein

Mix all the ingredients together in a blender and blend until smooth.

Pour in a nonstick pan and fry in medium heat until both sides look brown.

Putting all concepts together

Forty should not be the age for regrets, but rather a time to reflect on the future. Just daydreaming about doing something someday is not enough, nor should you accept the fact that you are out of shape or overweight. Taking action now, today, is a MUST if you genuinely want to improve and enjoy your life in the years to come.

Age should be a sign of success, not a signal of becoming weaker. Yes, physiologically, we are getting older, but this shouldn't deter anyone from making plans, be it in their career, health, family, or finances. You will begin to learn how to take better care of yourself and witness the miracles that the mind and body can accomplish.

In my twenty-five years of experience working with people who wanted to change their appearance and their lives—both men and women—I found that they all had one thing in common: the desire to transform their bodies. I saw that they had dreamt about it for a long time, perhaps for years. In some cases, excuses or real problems got in the way. But in the end, they did one thing: one day, they said, 'Enough is enough!' They made this life-changing decision and then took action.

Taking action was hard and uncomfortable, but persistence and determination took them a long way. You don't have to wait for people to applaud your change. This may never happen, at least not at first. However, later on, they will all admire your courage, your focus, and your dedication.

This is as much mental as it is physical. It's your state of mind that needs to be reset. All these men and women made incredible changes in their lives. Some had no real guidance on how to eat right, how to exercise, what to do, and for how long. Others sacrificed a lot of time, cut their sleep short, and, in the end, crossed the finishing line. As I mentioned, eating at the right time and consuming the right kind of foods is crucial. But adding regular exercise to this is the long-term solution.

Our bodies respond best to resistance training for building stronger muscles, bones, higher metabolism, better digestion and absorption of nutrients, and lower cholesterol, just to name a few.

The miracles of training provide excellent health with minimum risks of heart disease, diabetes, and osteoporosis.

People who incorporate training into their lives tend to enjoy better quality of life, more independence, greater mobility, and have fewer accidents.

By acting today, you will enjoy not only the body you always wanted, but great health and tremendous energy.

Now you have the tools. Enjoy your transformation!

To contact me or for training and nutrition consultation please visit: https://www.catherinepiotinstitute.com.

Section 3

EXERCISE GUIDE

Exercise 1: Incline chest press

Start Position:

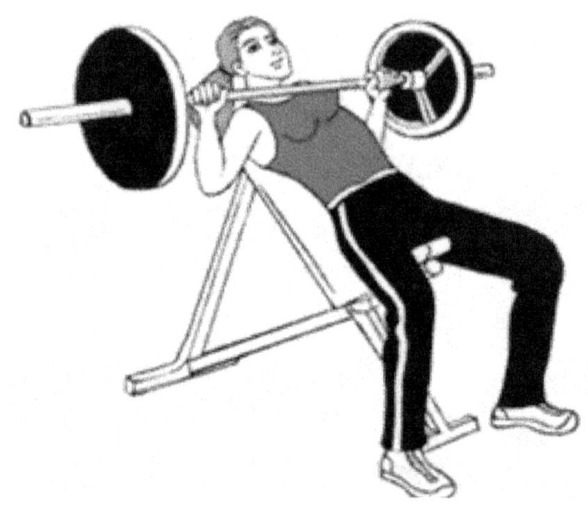

Finish Position:

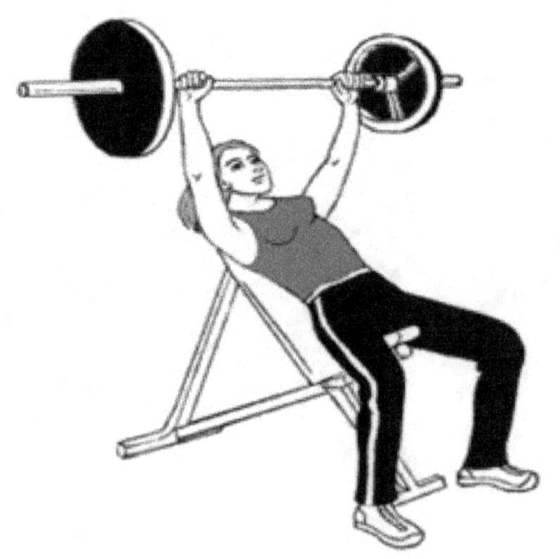

Exercise 2: Chest bench press

Start Position:

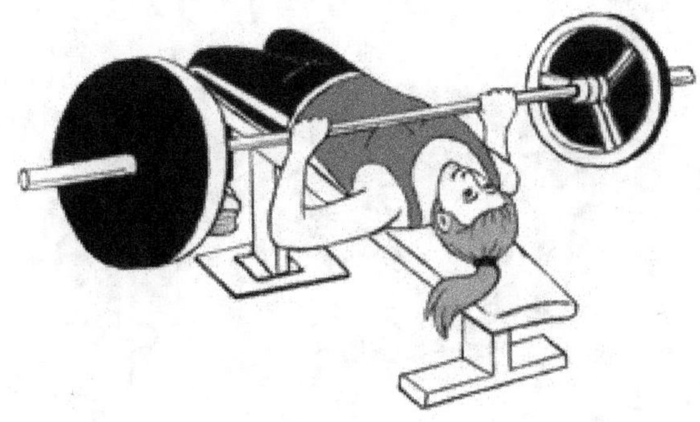

Finish Position:

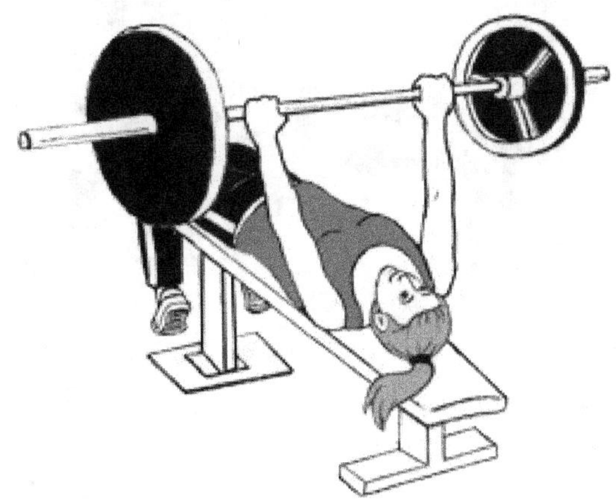

Exercise 3: Chest flyes

Start Position:

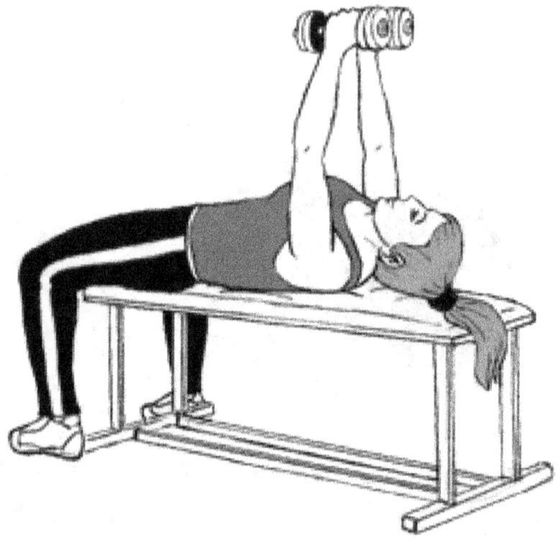

Finish Position:

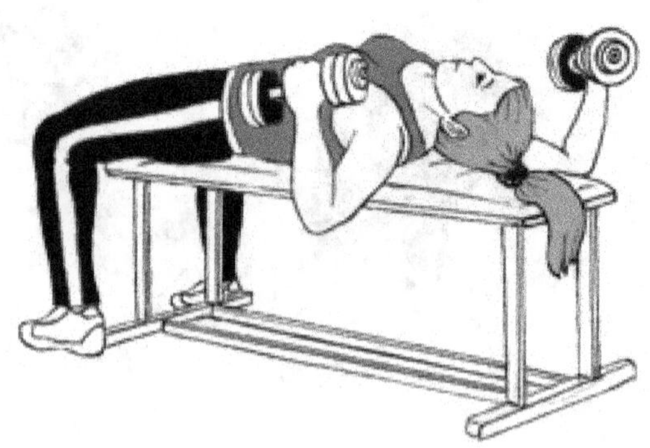

Exercise 4: Chest press with dumbbells

Start Position:

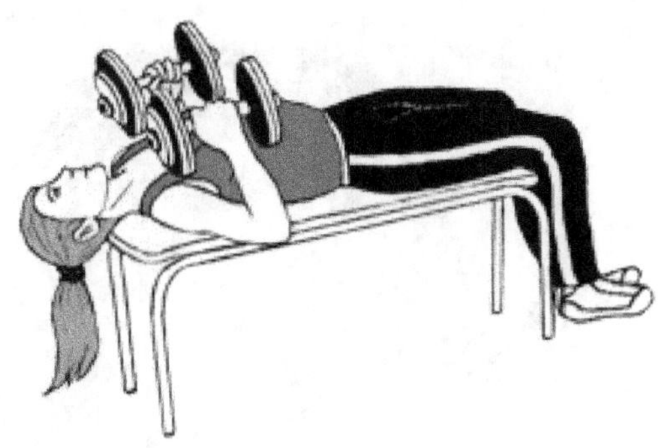

Finish Position:

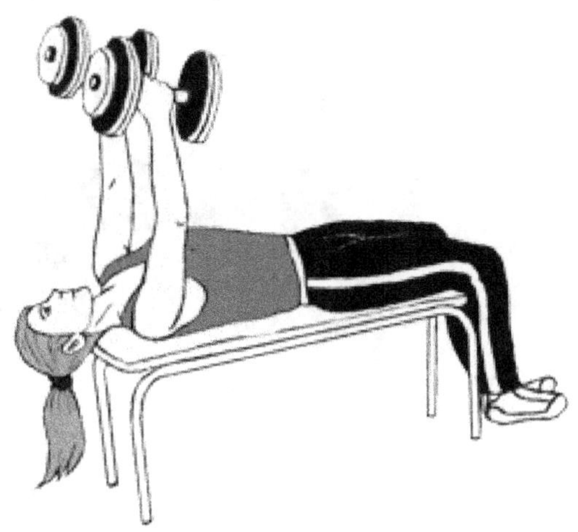

Exercise 5: Pullover upper chest

Start Position:

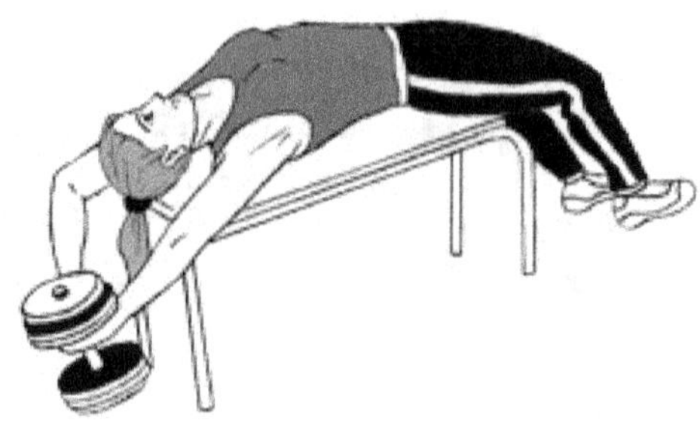

Finish Position:

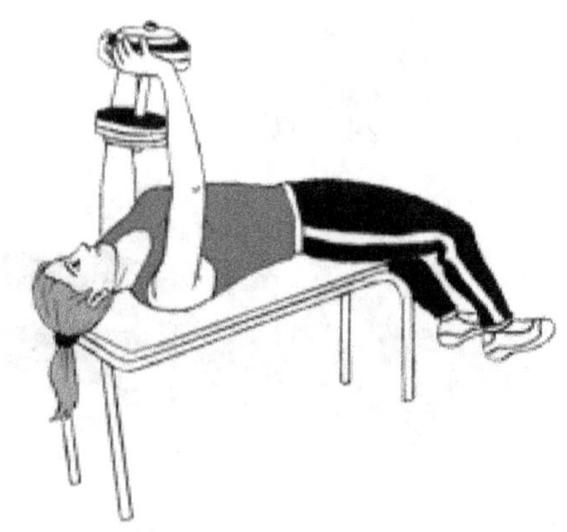

Exercise 6: Push-up

Start Position:

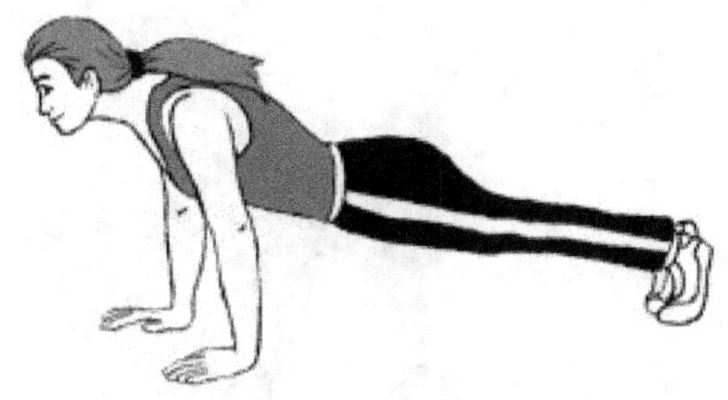

Finish Position:

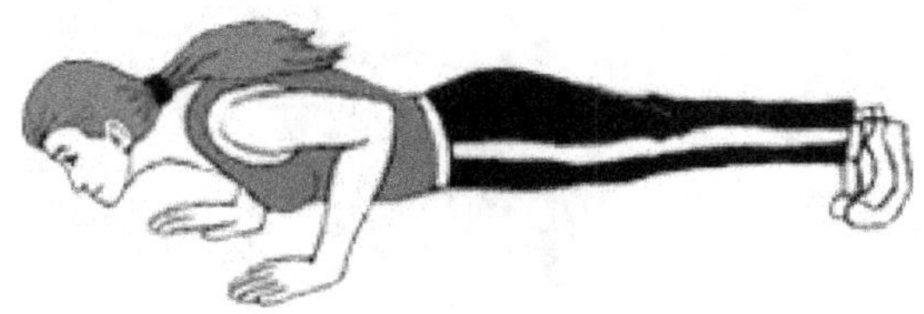

Exercise 7: Shoulders press with dumbbells

Start Position:

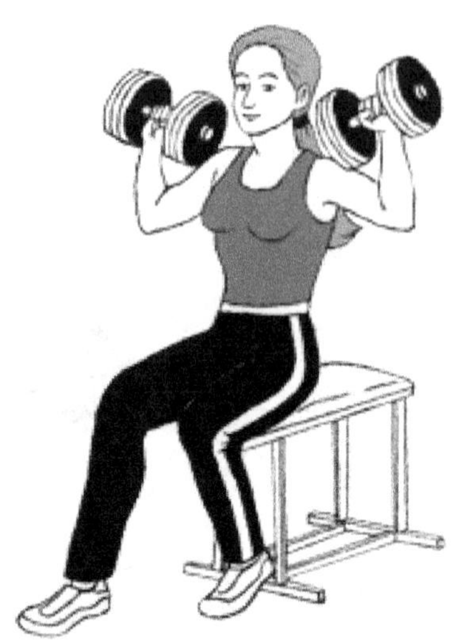

Finish Position:

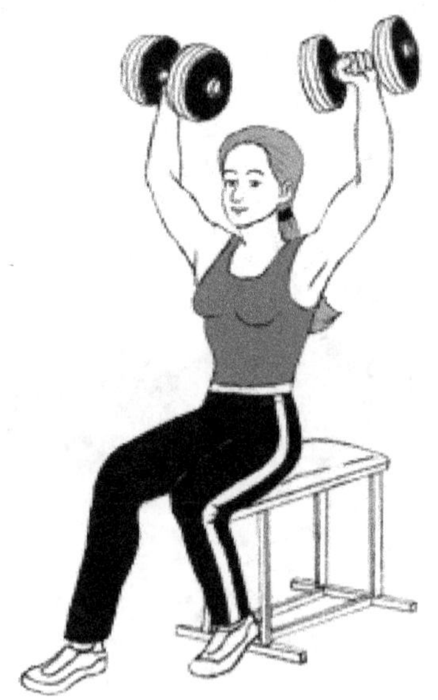

Exercise 8: Shoulder press alternating

Start Position:

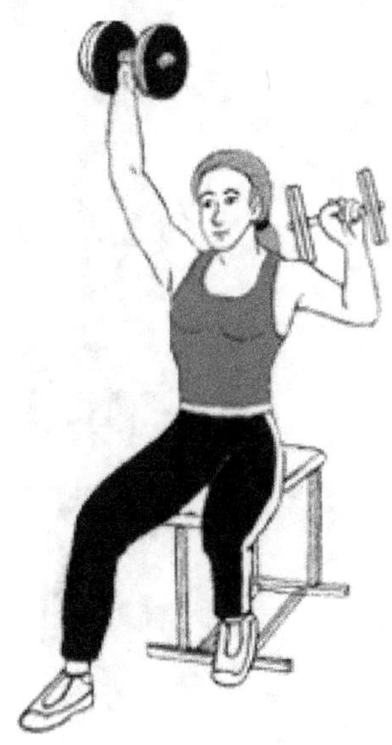

Finish Position:

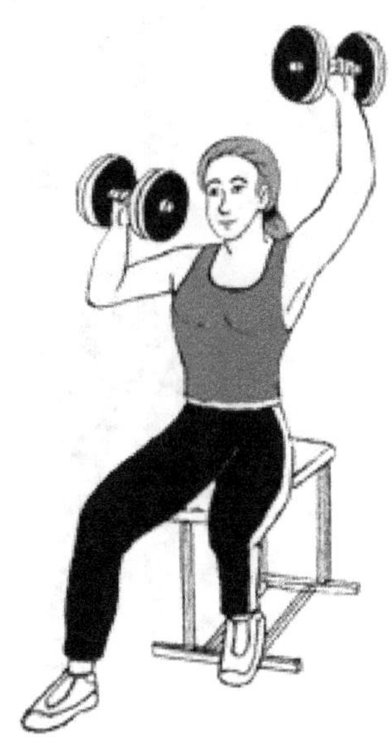

Exercise 9: Shoulders upright row with dumbbells

Start Position:

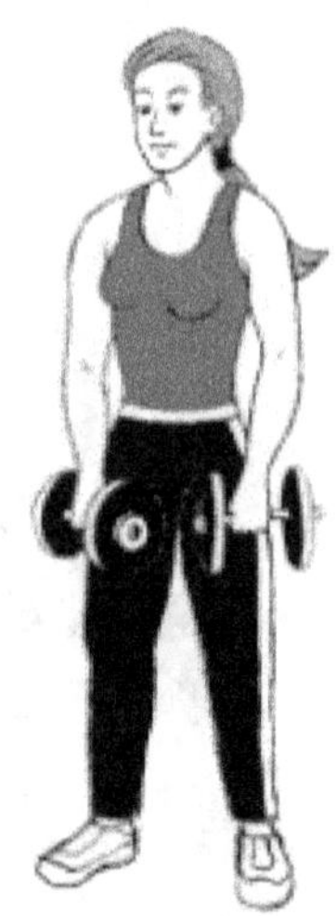

Finish Position:

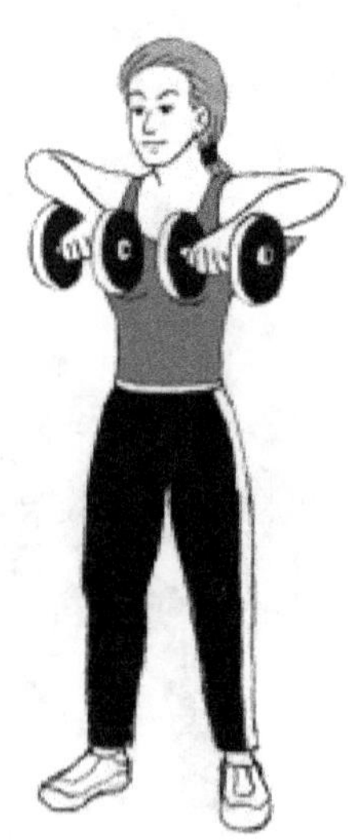

Exercise 10: Shoulders front raise with barbell

Start Position:

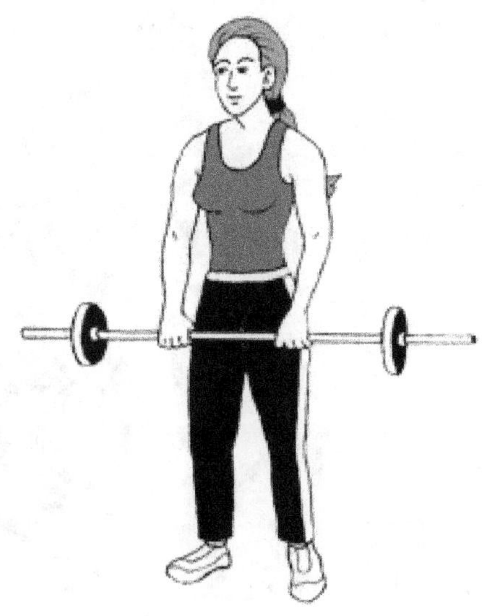

Finish Position:

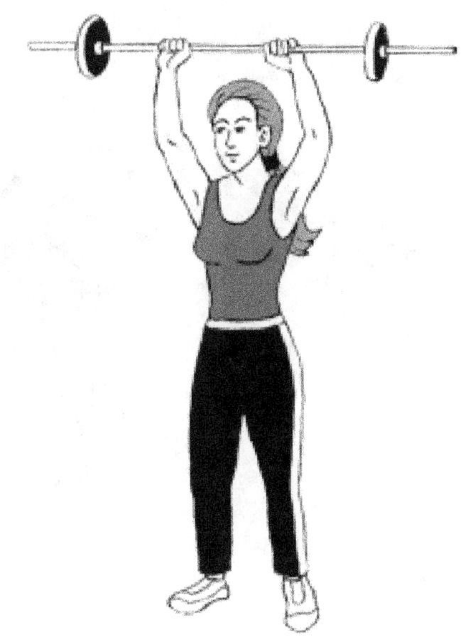

Exercise 11: Shoulders – Front raise

Start Position:

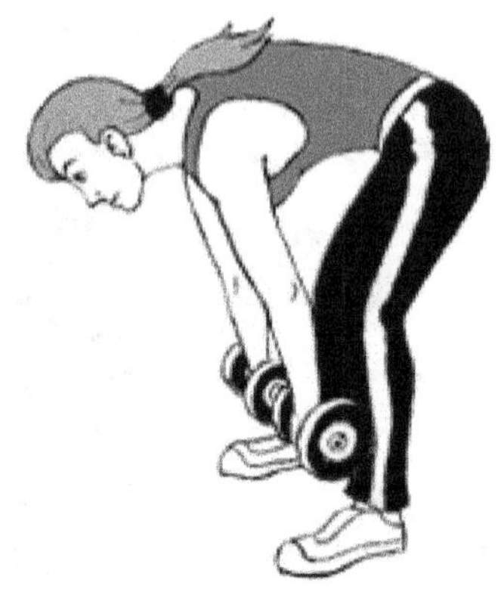

Finish Position:

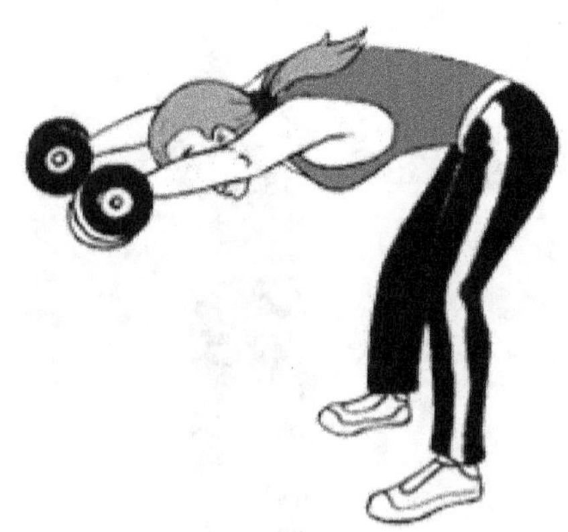

Exercise 12: Shoulders one arm bent over lateral raise

Start Position:

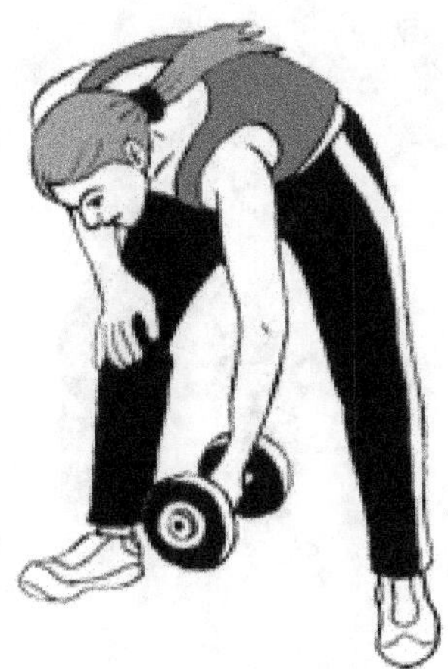

Finish Position:

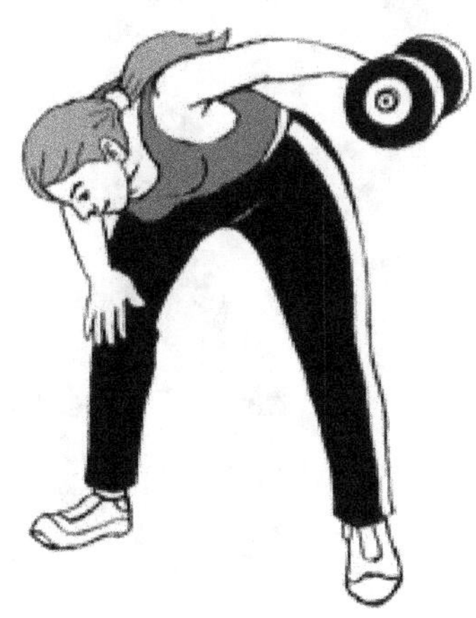

Exercise 13: Shoulder press with barbell

Start Position:

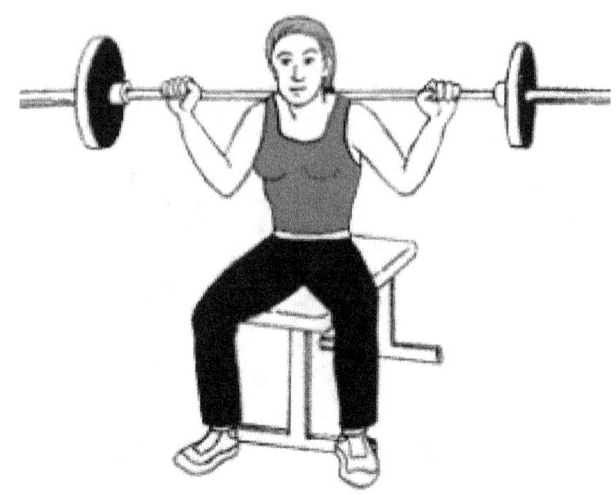

Finish Position:

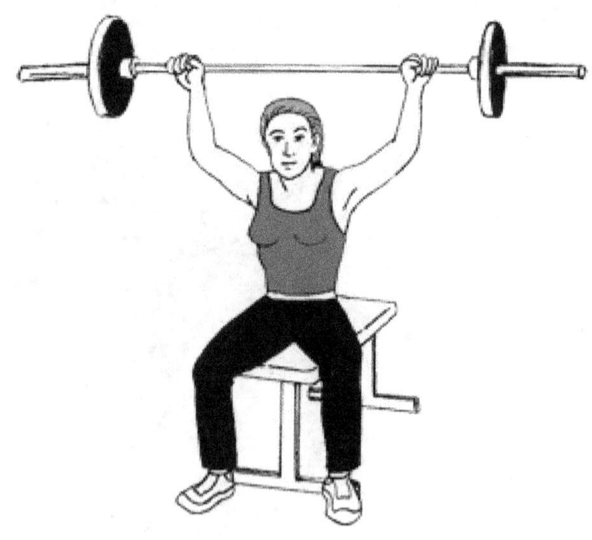

Exercise 14: Shoulders – Military press

Start Position:

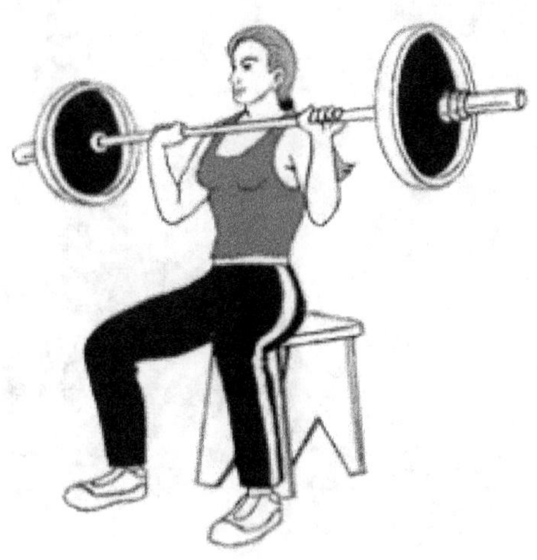

Finish Position:

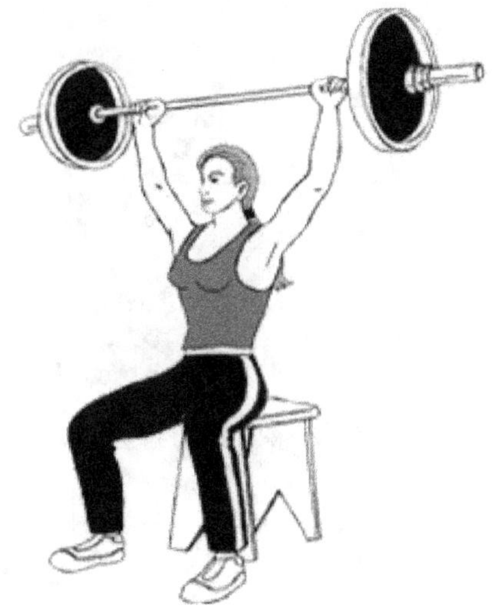

Exercise 15: Shoulders-sited lateral raise

Start Position:

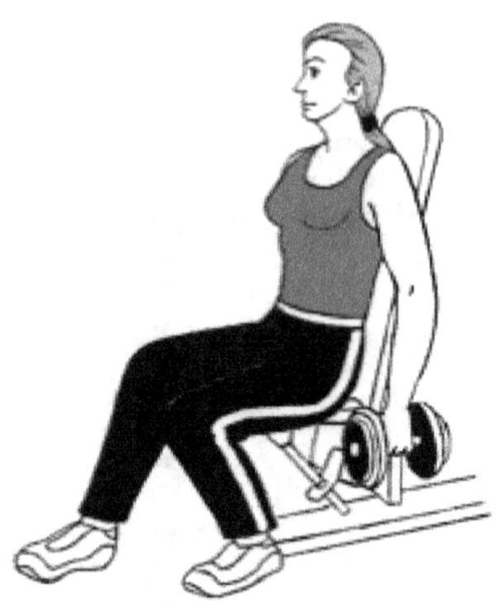

Finish Position:

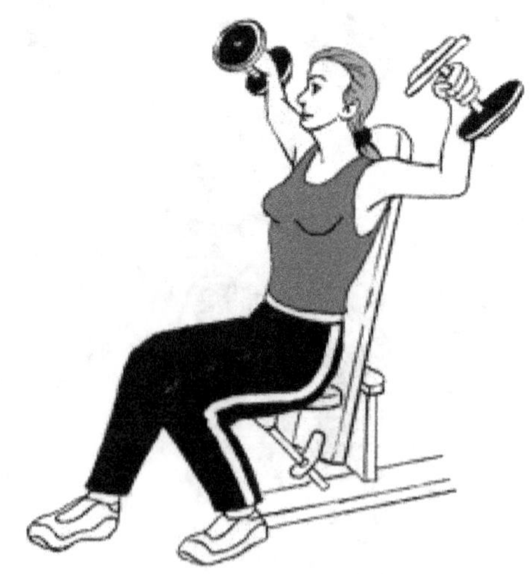

Exercise 16: Shoulders-standing lateral raise

Start Position:

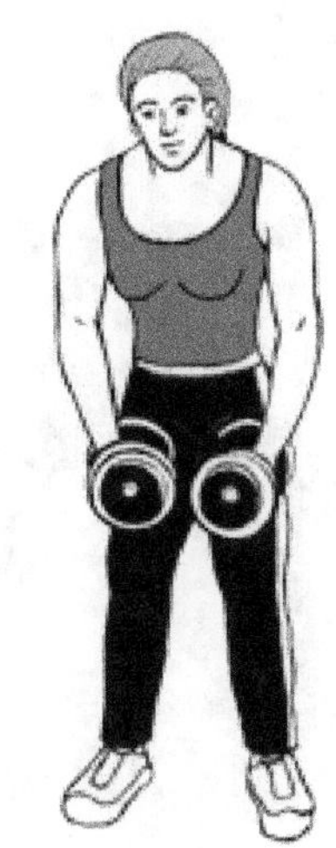

Finish Position:

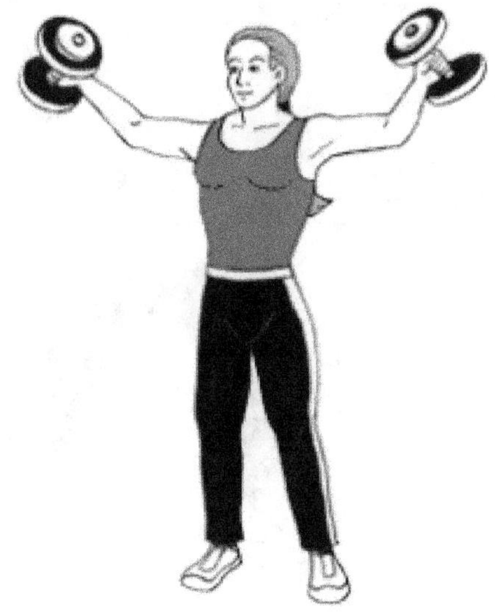

Exercise 17: Shoulders-bent over cable lateral raise

Start Position:

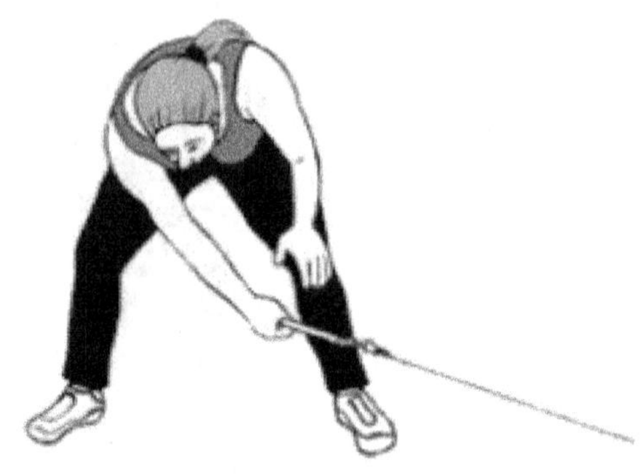

Finish Position:

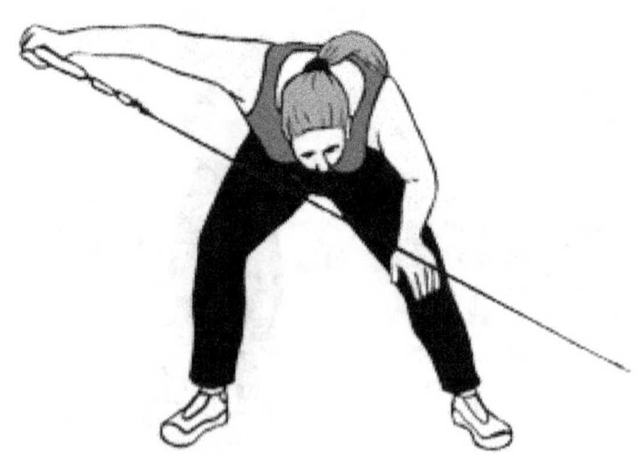

Exercise 18: Shoulders-cable upright row

Start Position:

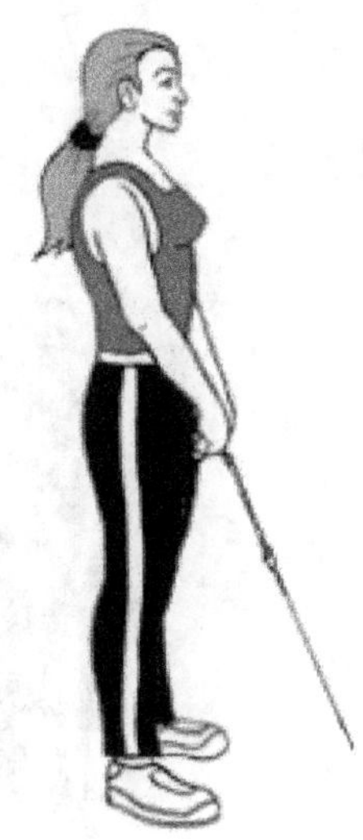

Finish Position:

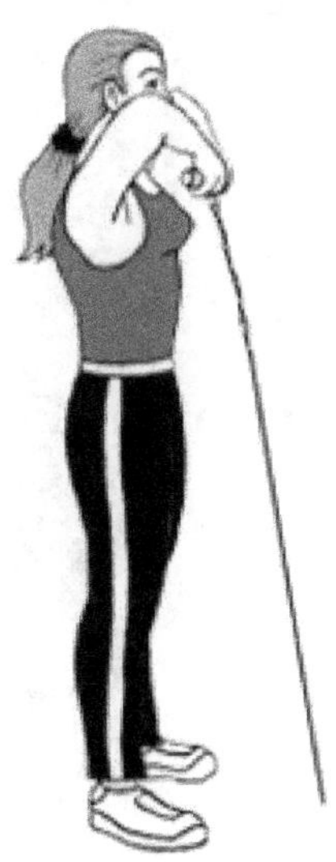

Exercise 19: Back-pull down front

Start Position:

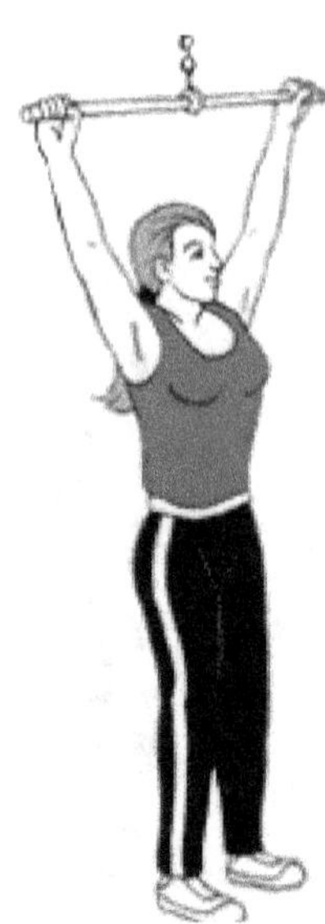

Finish Position:

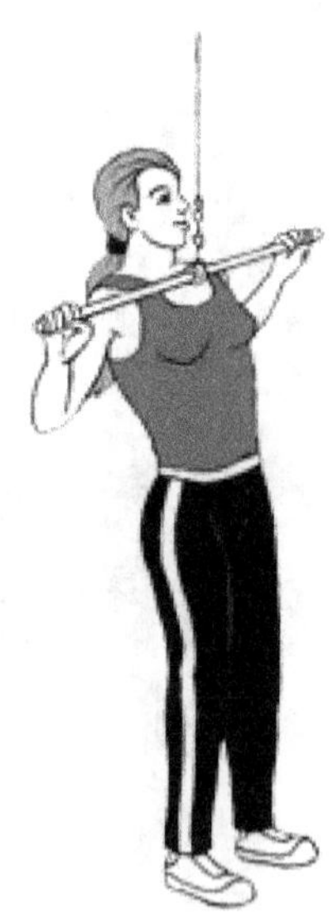

Exercise 20: Back-reverse close grip pull down

Start Position:

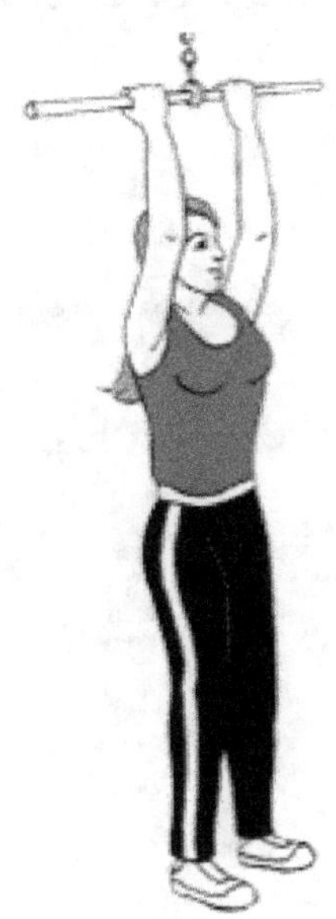

Finish Position:

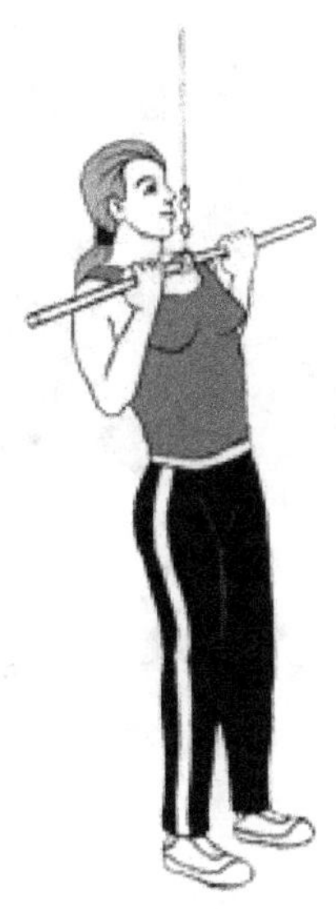

Exercise 21: Back-barbell bent over row

Start Position:

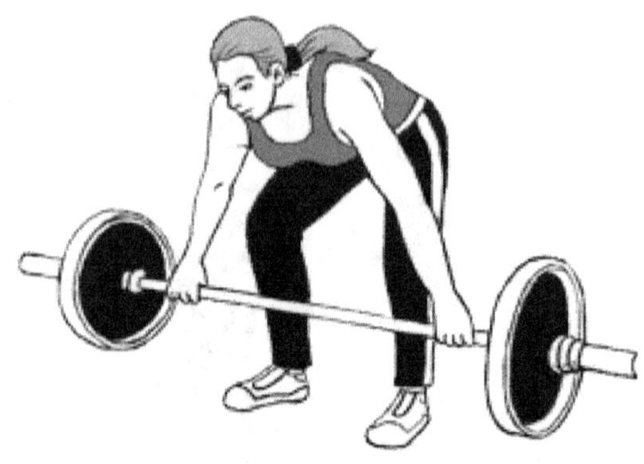

Finish Position:

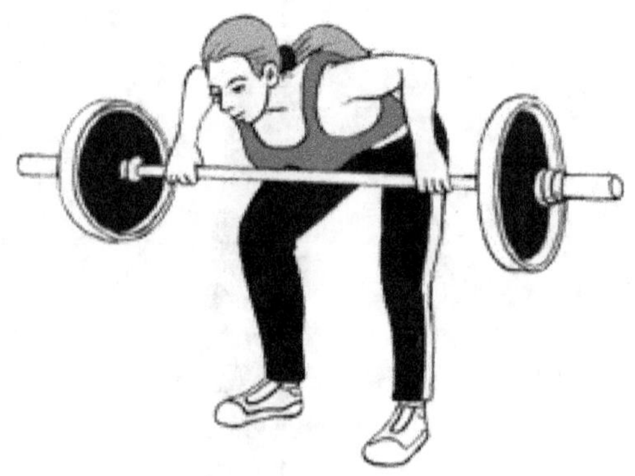

Exercise 22: Back-one arm dumbbell row

Start Position:

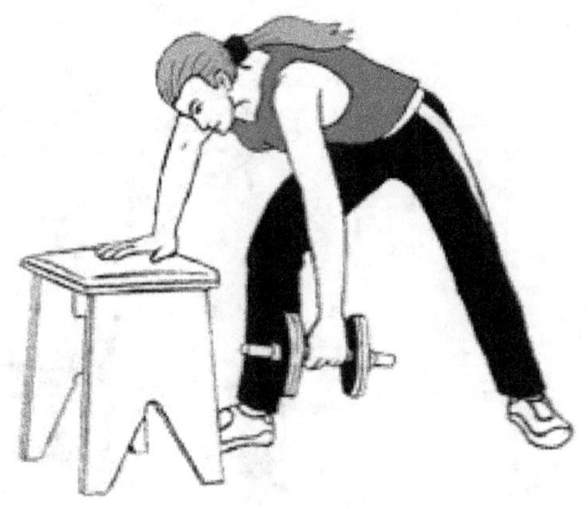

Finish Position:

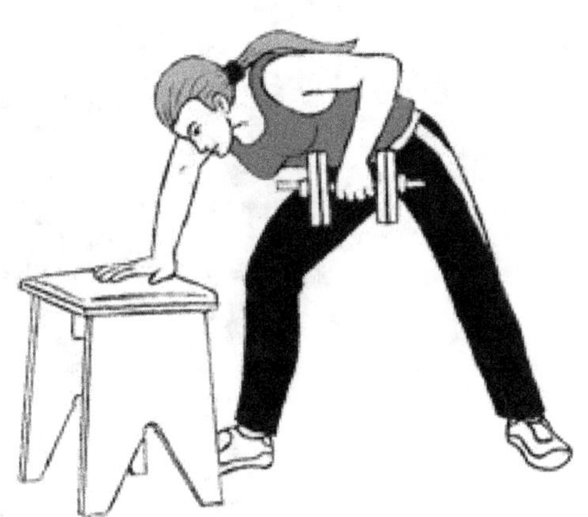

Exercise 23: Back-T-bar row

Start Position:

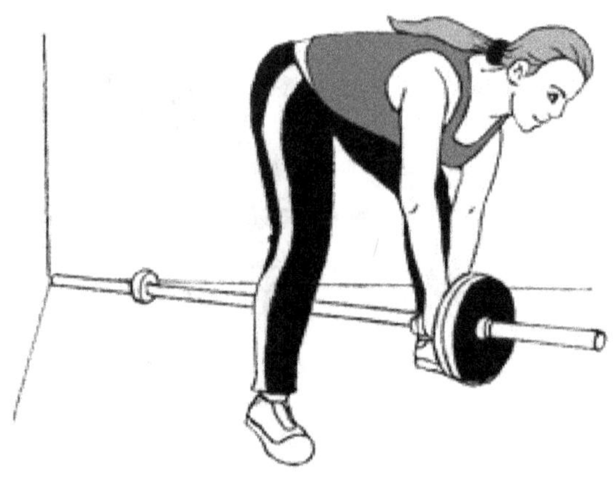

Finish Position:

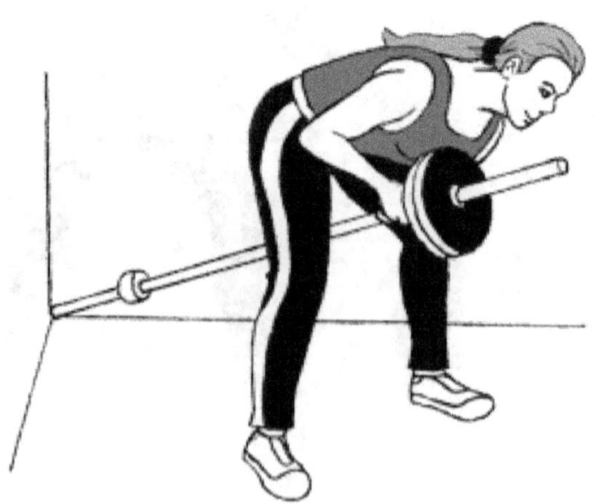

Exercise 24: Back-sited close grip cable row

Start Position:

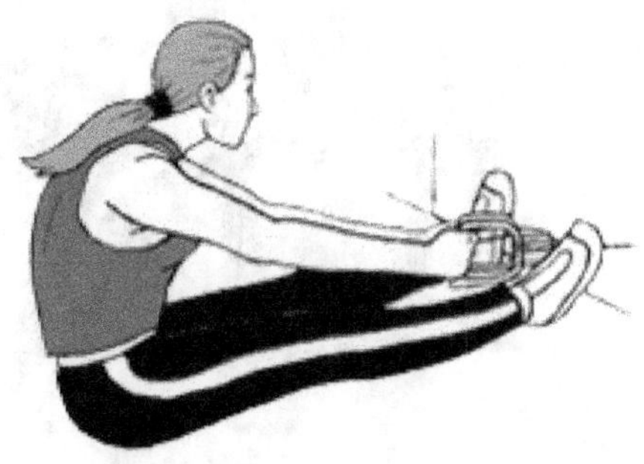

Finish Position:

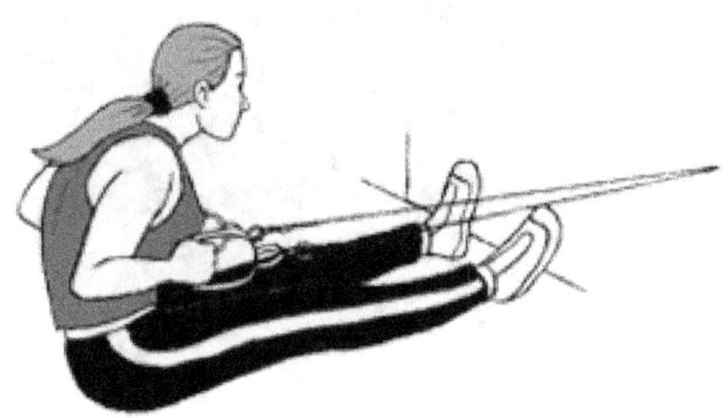

Exercise 25: Triceps-one arm triceps extension

Start Position:

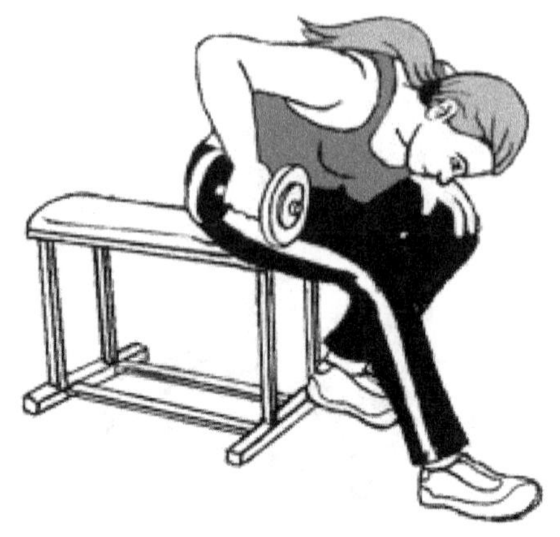

Finish Position:

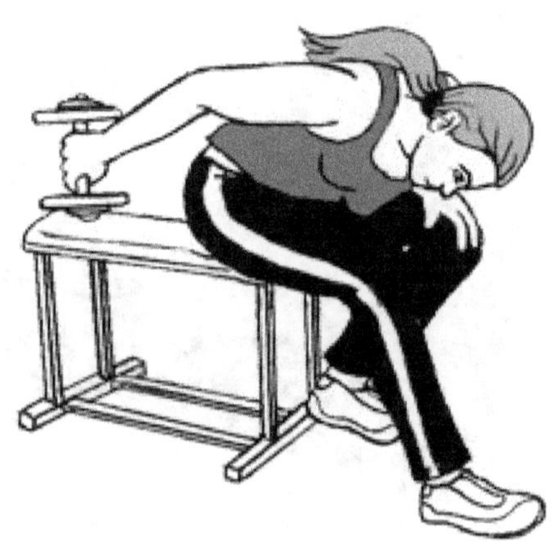

Exercise 26: Triceps extension

Start Position:

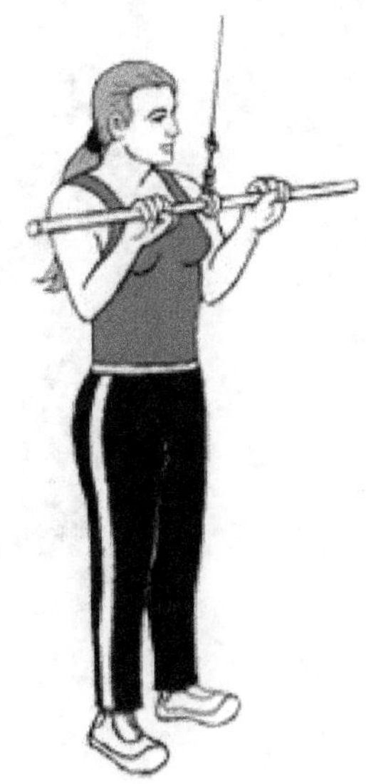

Finish Position:

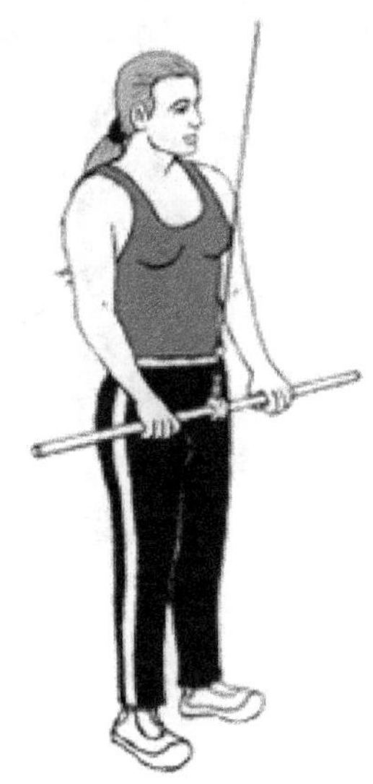

Exercise 27: Triceps extension reverse grip

Start Position:

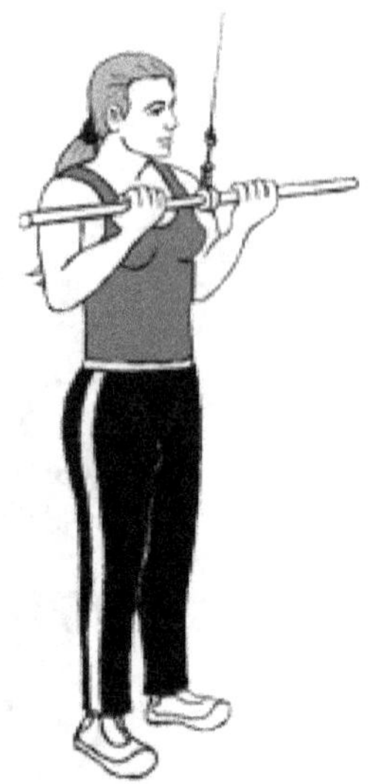

Finish Position:

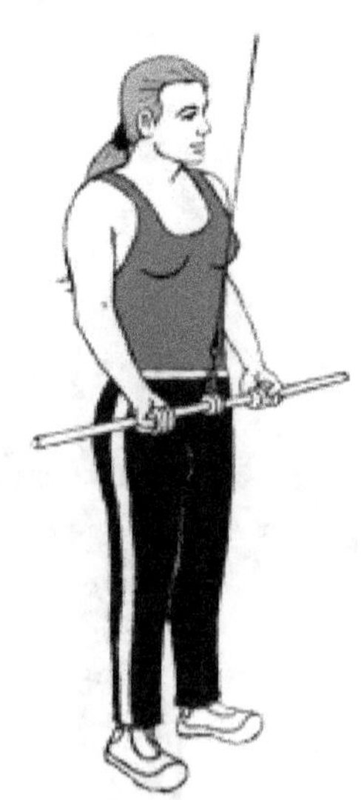

Exercise 28: Biceps curl with barbell

Start Position:

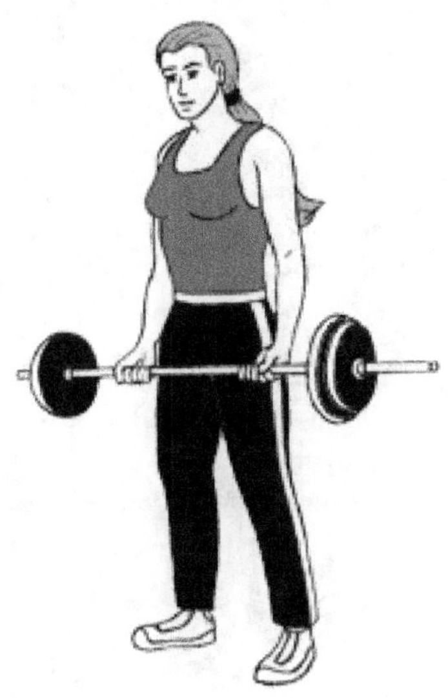

Finish Position:

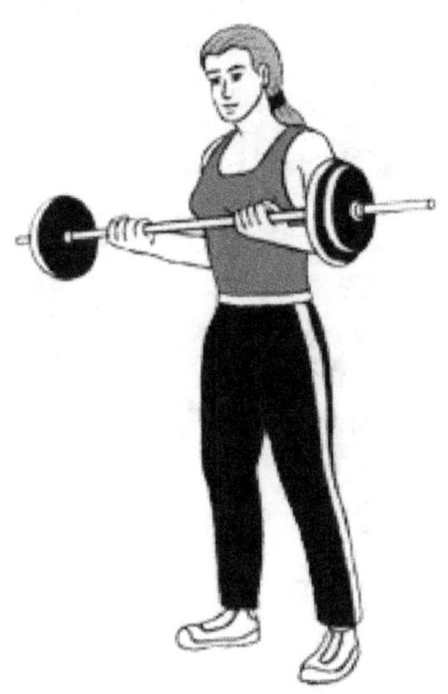

Exercise 29: Biceps curl with cable

Start Position:

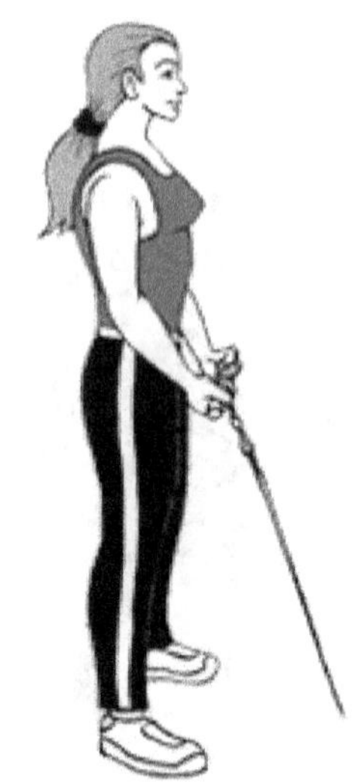

Finish Position:

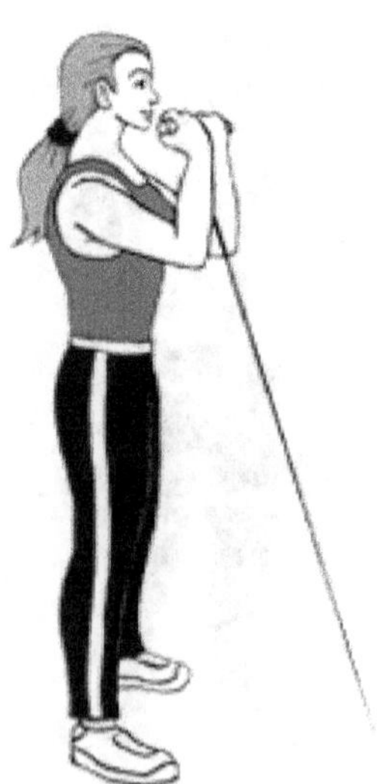

Exercise 30: Biceps curl with dumbbell alternating

Start Position:

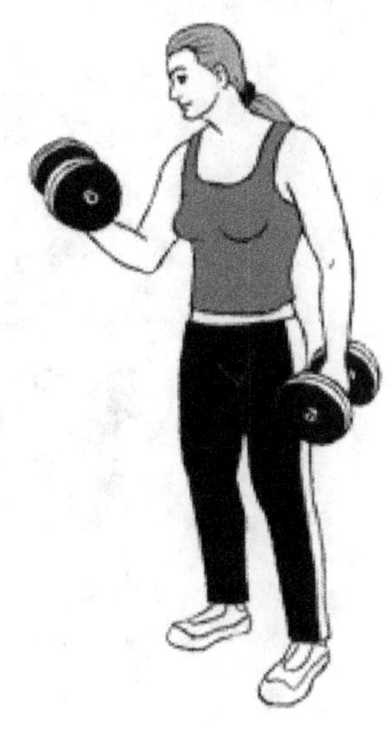

Finish Position:

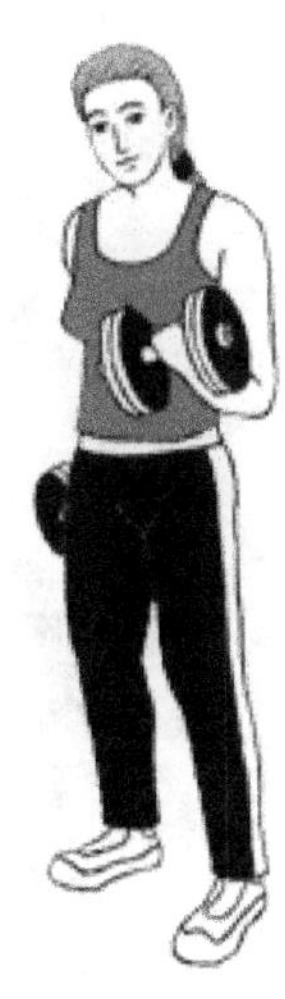

Exercise 31: Biceps concentration curl

Start Position:

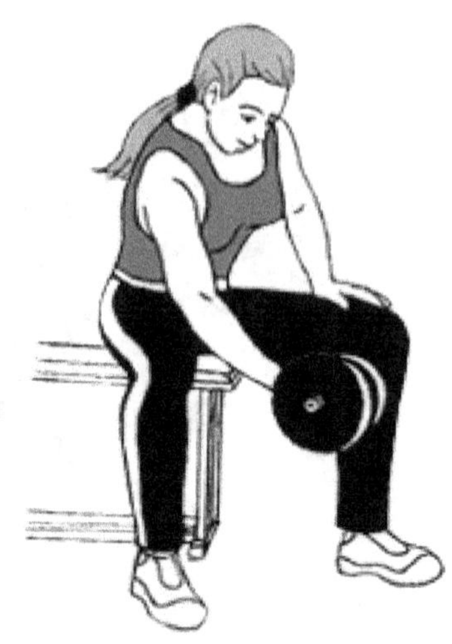

Finish Position:

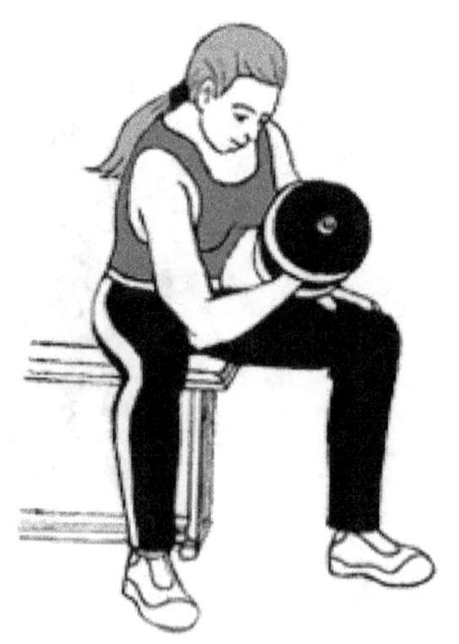

Exercise 32: Legs-dead lift

Start Position:

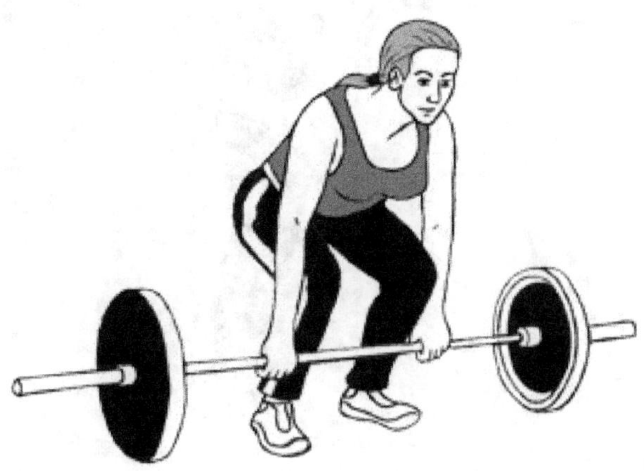

Finish Position:

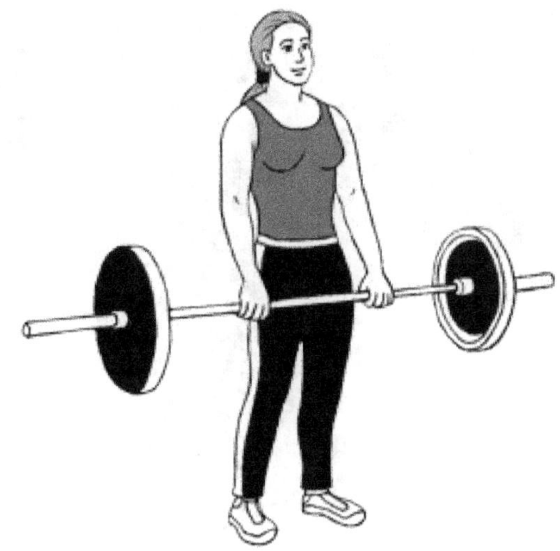

Exercise 33: Legs-squat

Start Position:

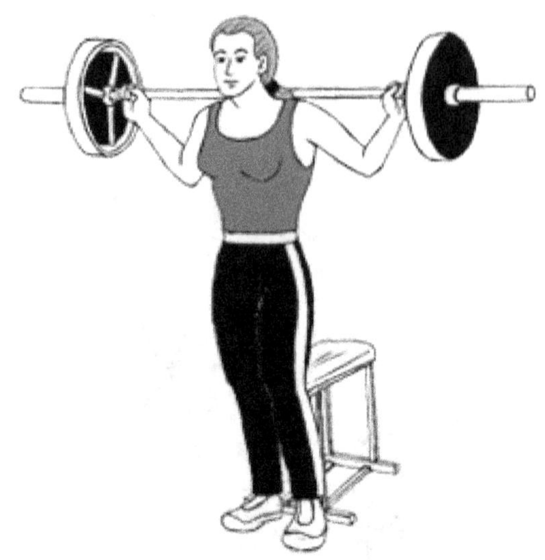

Finish Position:

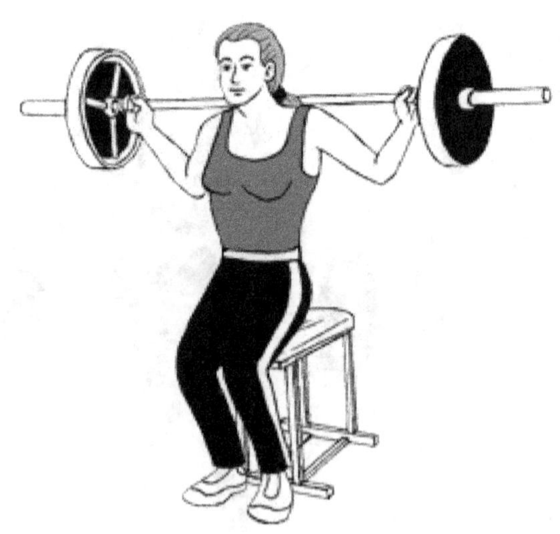

Exercise 34: Legs-press

Start Position:

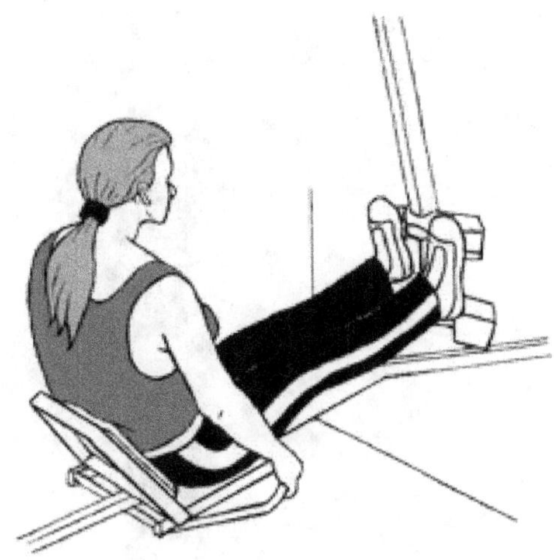

Finish Position:

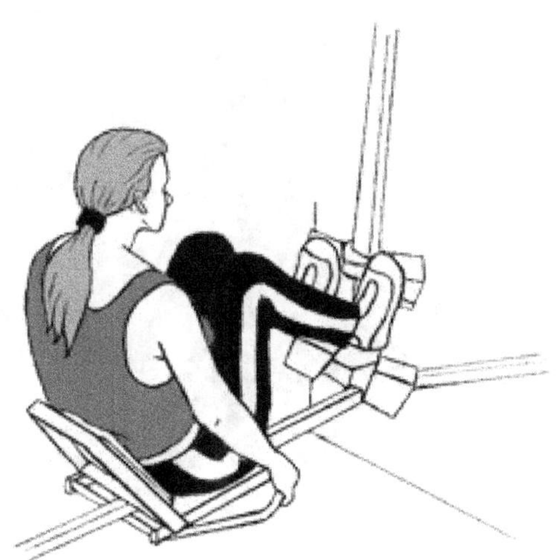

Exercise 35: Legs–back lunge

Start Position:

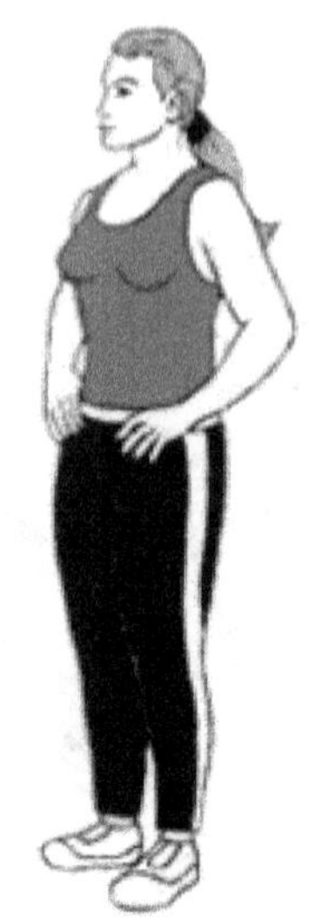

Finish Position:

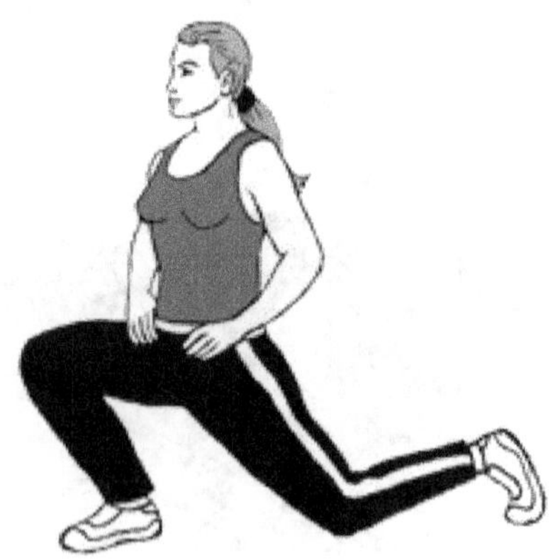

Exercise 36: Legs-front lunge with barbell

Start Position:

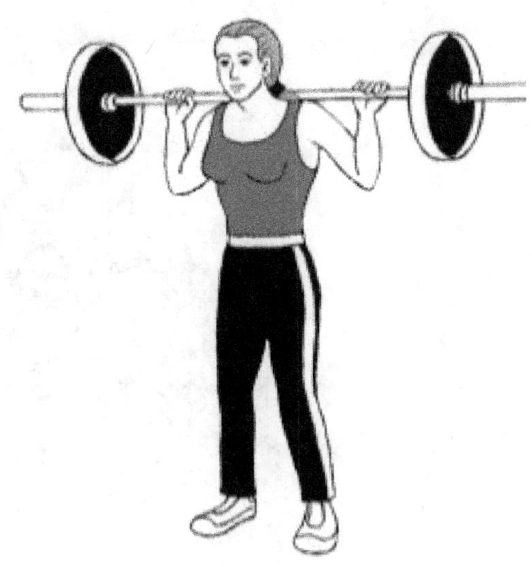

Finish Position:

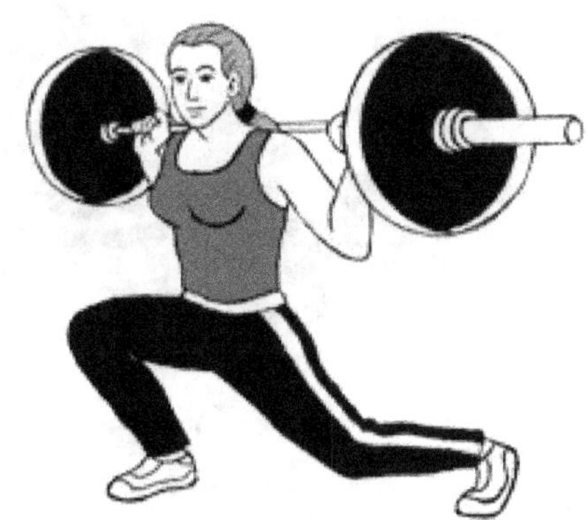

Exercise 37: Legs-extension

Start Position:

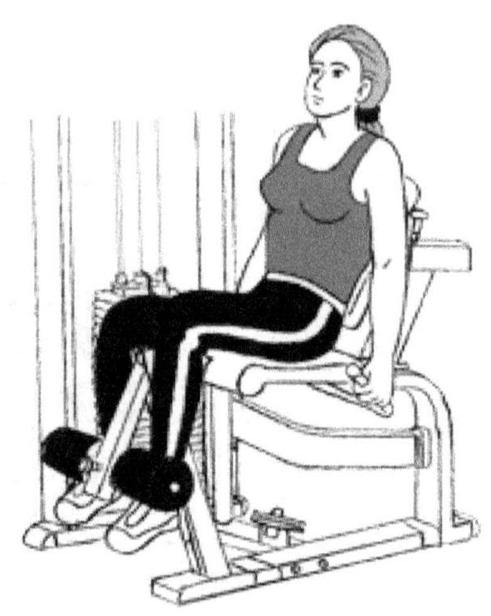

Finish Position:

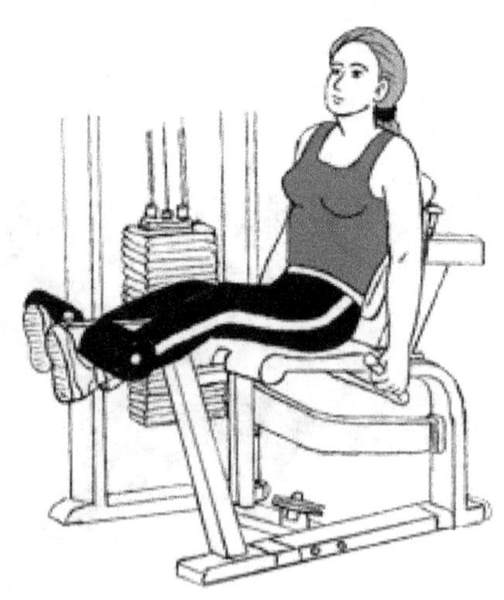

Exercise 38: Legs-hamstring curl

Start Position:

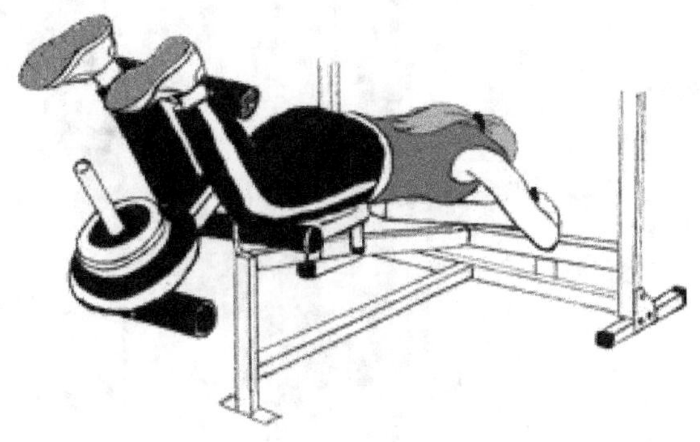

Finish Position:

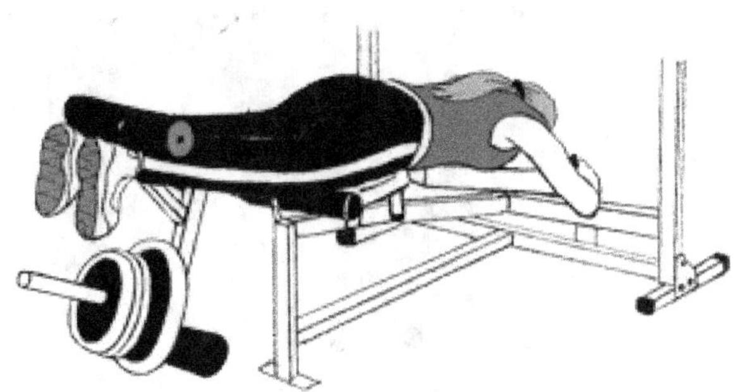

Exercise 39: Legs-adduction

Start Position:

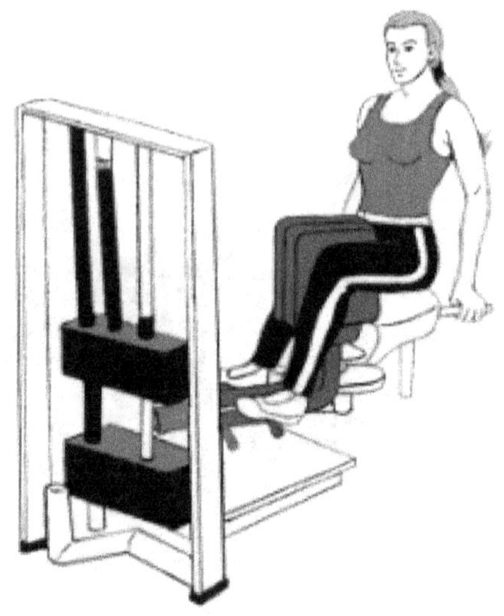

Finish Position:

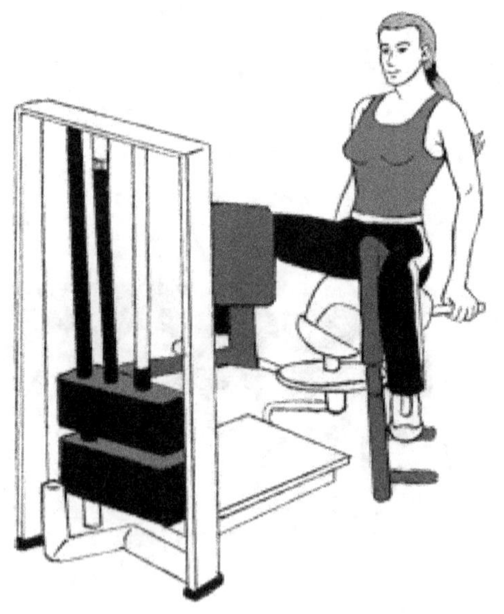

Exercise 40: Back-Lower Back extension

Start Position:

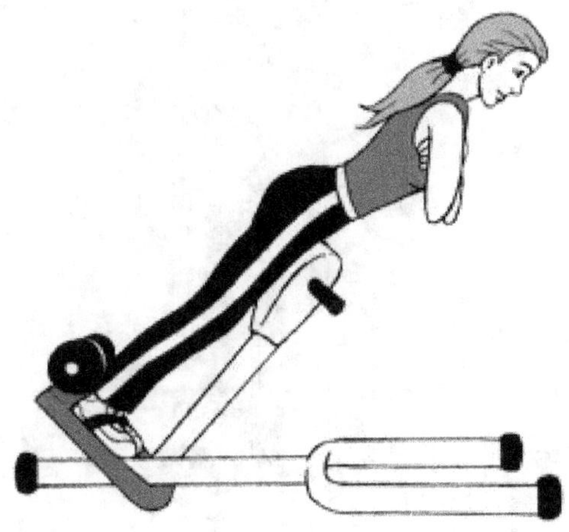

Finish Position:

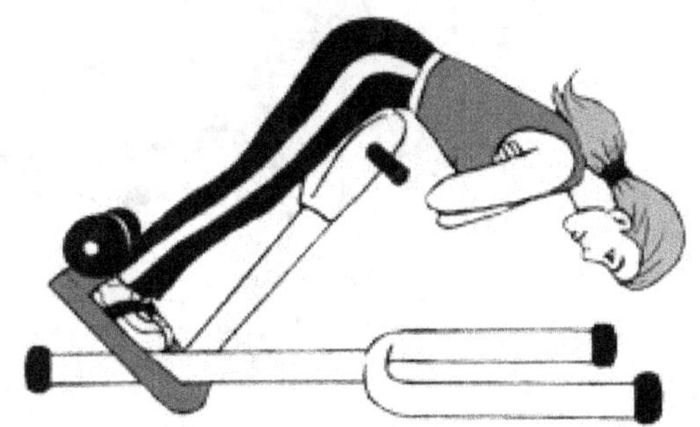

Exercise 41: Legs-kick back

Start Position:

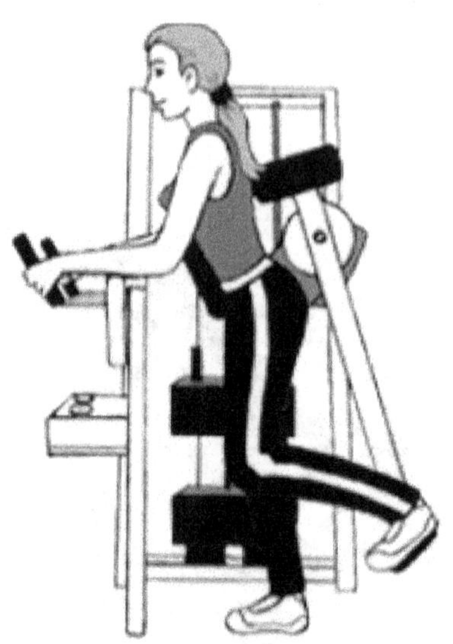

Finish Position:

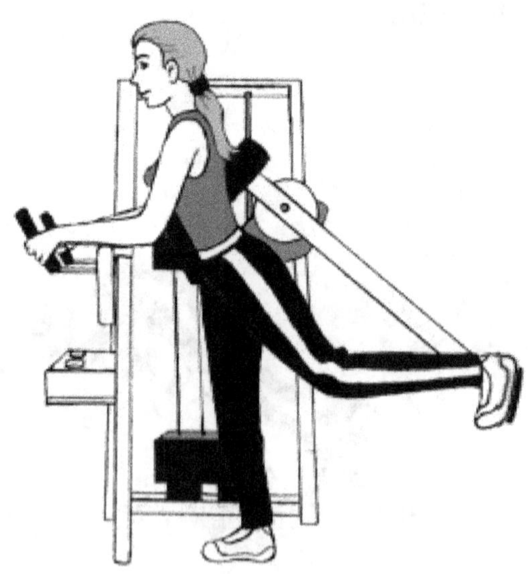

Exercise 42: Legs-cable kickback

Start Position:

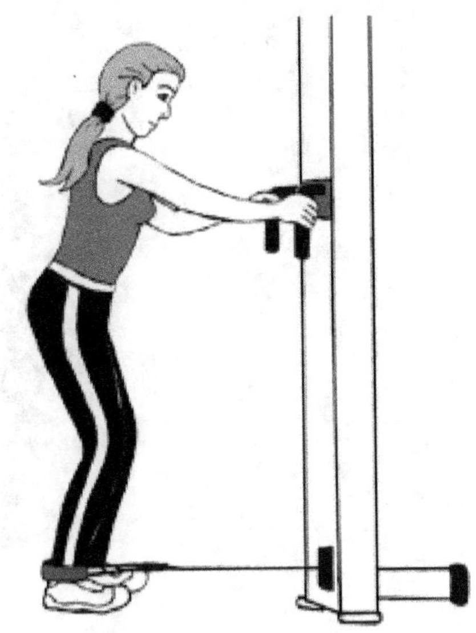

Finish Position:

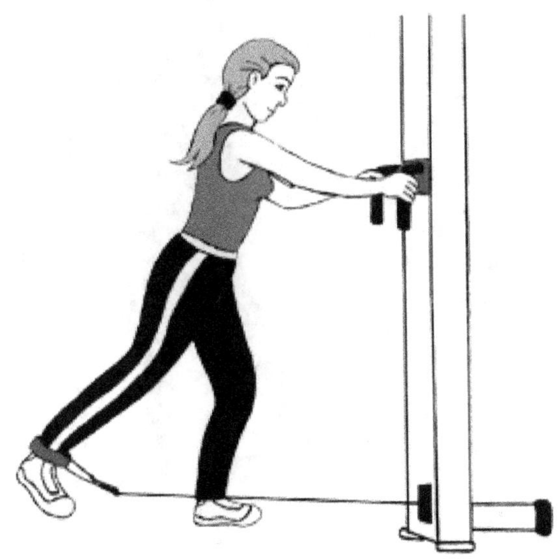

Exercise 43: Legs-cable abduction

Start Position:

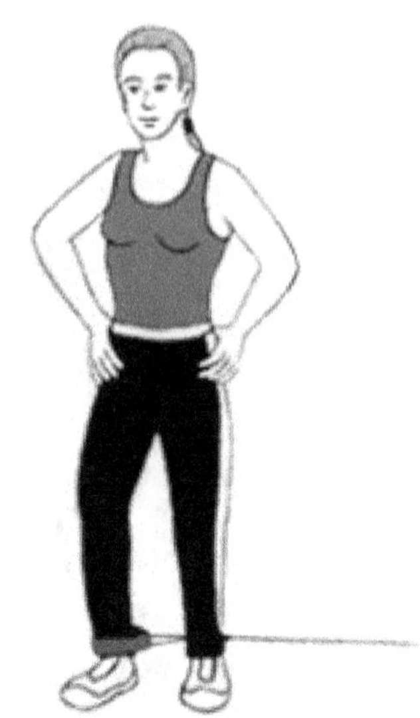

Finish Position:

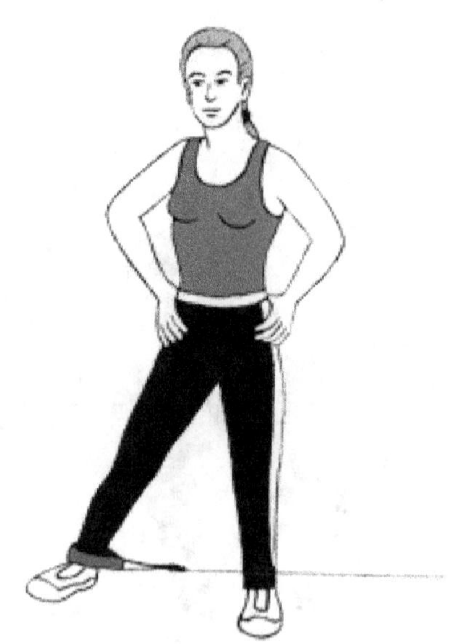

Exercise 44: Legs-hack squat

Start Position:

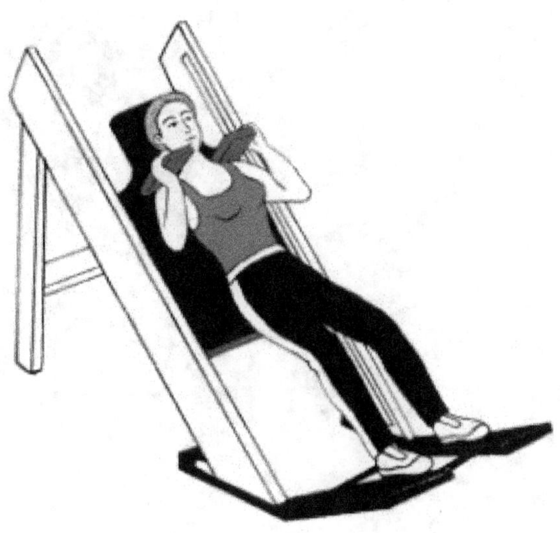

Finish Position:

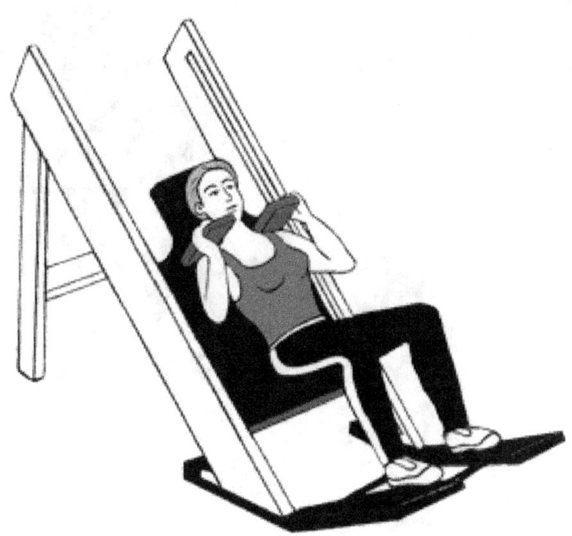

Exercise 45: Legs-calves press

Start Position:

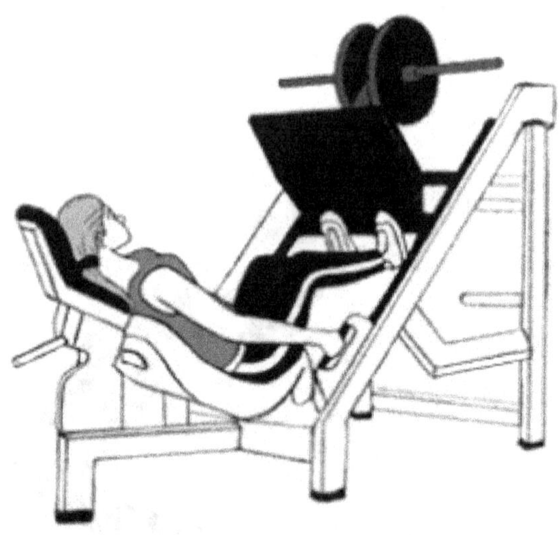

Finish Position:

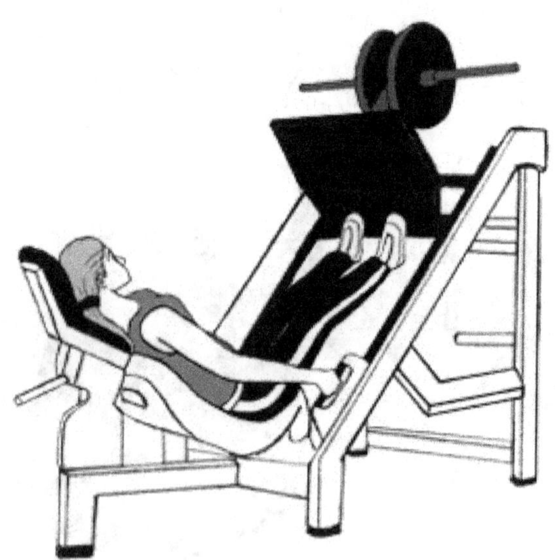

Exercise 46: Legs-adduction

Start Position:

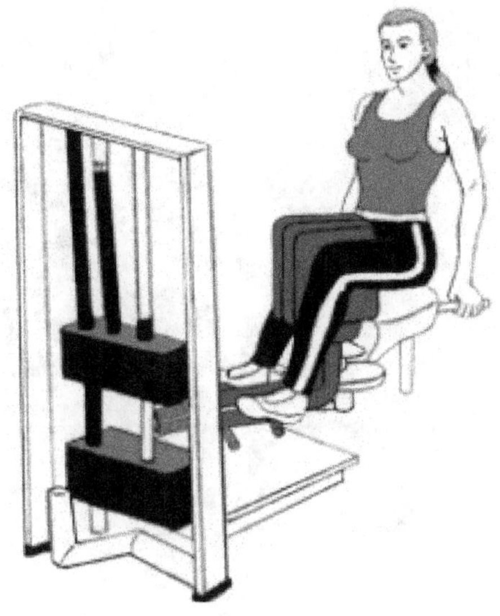

Finish Position:

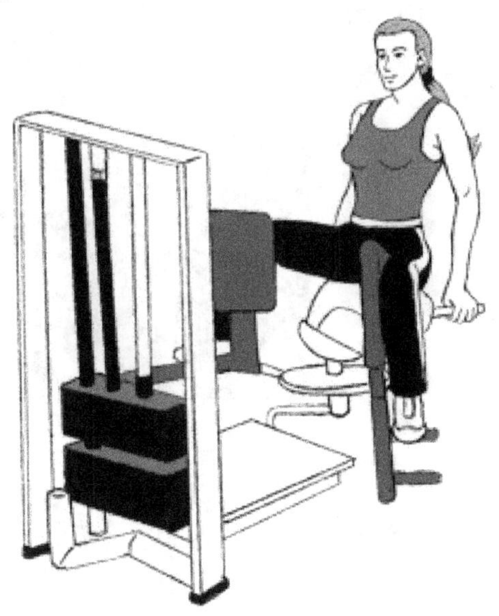

Exercise 47: Abs-twisted crunches

Start Position:

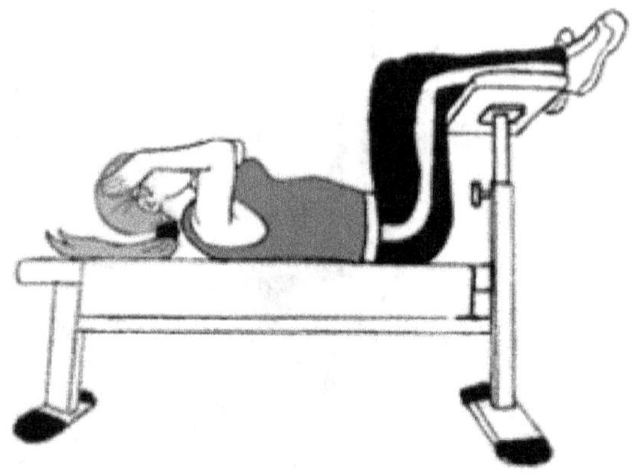

Finish Position:

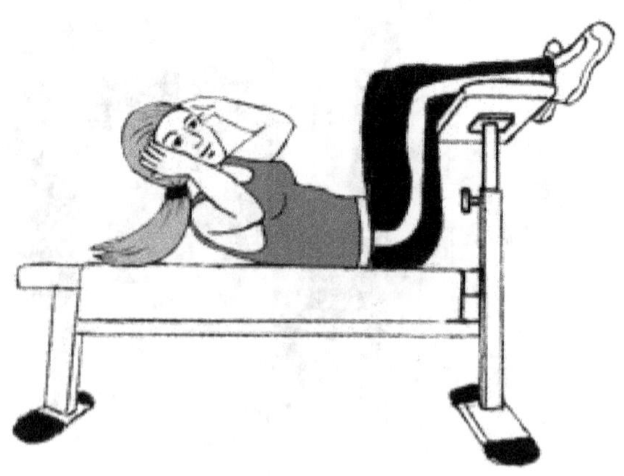

Exercise 48: Abs-knee up

Start Position:

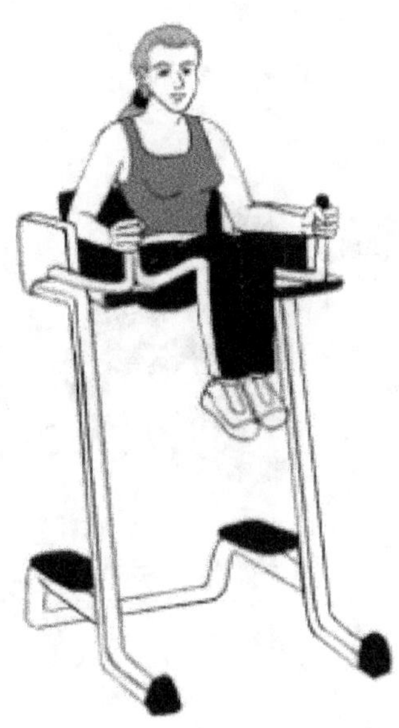

Finish Position:

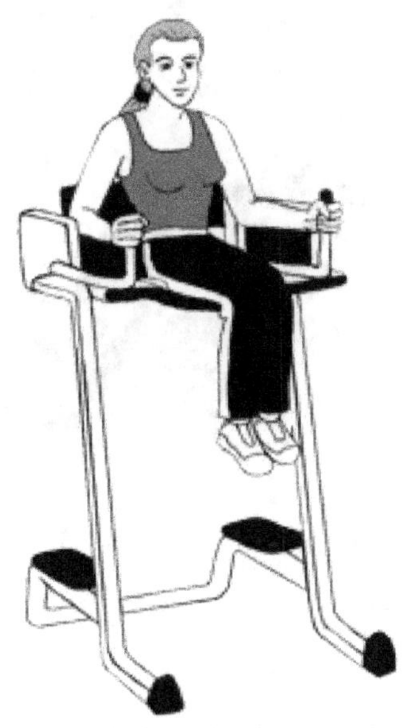

Exercise 49: Abs-machine crunches

Start Position:

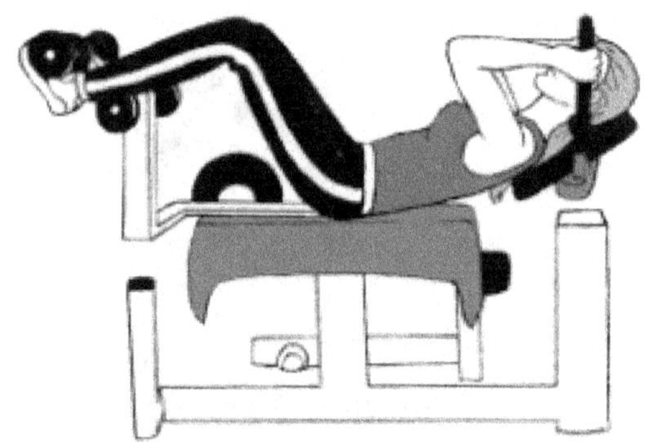

Finish Position:

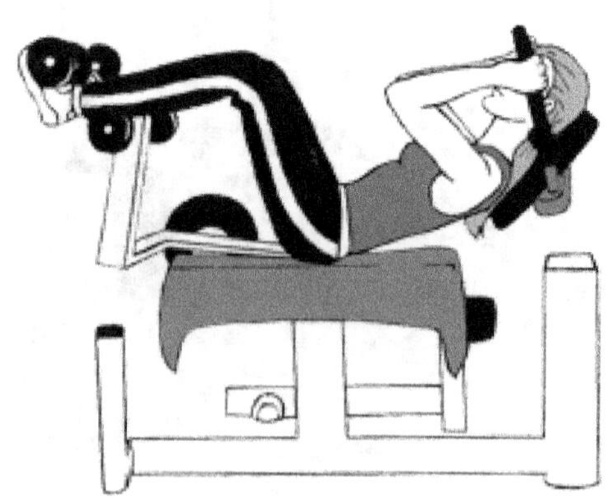

Conclusion

Congratulations on completing this book! I hope you had a blast reading it!

Now, get ready to dive into the information and practical tips that will kickstart your journey to a transformed leaner, healthier and fitter you!

Make sure you grab the exclusive free gift (link below) if you haven't already. It's a game-changer!

https://bit.ly/free-healthyeatingguide

Oh, and before you go, I'd absolutely love to hear your thoughts. Leave a review and let me know what you love or what I can do better, it would be great to hear from you.

Calling all amazing women who are determined to shed those extra pounds and transform their bodies and lifestyles! Let's connect for a free consultation (link below).

https://calendly.com/catherinepiot

Together, we'll discuss your goals and map out your path to success. Let's make it happen!

https://catherinepiotinstitute.com

https://facebook.com/catherinepiot

https://instagram.com/catherinepiot.tv

www.ingramcontent.com/pod-product-compliance
Lightning Source LLC
Chambersburg PA
CBHW050811260726
48660CB00004B/1369